Clinical Practice Management for Speech-Language Pathologists

Becky Sutherland Cornett, PhD
Director
Hospital Administration
The Ohio State University Medical Center
Columbus, Ohio

Library of Congress Cataloging-in-Publication Data

Clinical practice management for speech-language pathologists /
edited by Becky Sutherland Cornett.
p. cm.—(Excellence in practice series)
Includes bibliographical references and index.
ISBN 0-8342-1094-0 (alk. paper)
1. Speech therapy—Practice. I. Cornett, Becky Sutherland. II. Series.
[DNLM: 1. Outcome Assessment (Health Care). 2. Practice Management, Medical.
3. Speech-Language Pathology—organization & administration. WL 340.2 C6414 1999]
RC428.5.C57 1999
616.85'5'0068—dc21
DNLM/DLC
for Library of Congress
99-21827
CIP

For information, address Aspen Publishers, Inc., Permissions Department,
200 Orchard Ridge Drive, Suite 200, Gaithersburg, Maryland 20878.

Orders: (800) 638-8437
Customer Service: (800) 234-1660

Editorial Services: Nora Fitzpatrick
Library of Congress Catalog Card Number: 99-21827
ISBN: 0-8342-1094-0

Printed in the United States of America

1 2 3 4 5

For my parents

Betty Jory Sutherland
(1924–1997)

Bruce A. Sutherland
(1924–1988)

Rest in peace

Table of Contents

Contributors

EDITOR

Becky Sutherland Cornett, PhD
Director, Hospital Administration
The Ohio State University Medical Center
Columbus, Ohio

CONTRIBUTORS

Noma B. Anderson, PhD
Associate Professor and Department Chair, Department of Communication Sciences and Disorders
Howard University
Washington, DC

Shelly S. Chabon, PhD
Associate Professor and Department Chair
Department of Communication Sciences and Disorders
Rockhurst College
Kansas City, Missouri

Tracy L. Davidson, MS
Program Director
Northland Terrace Medical Center
Columbus, Ohio

James Feeney, MS
Assistant Director, Speech Pathology
Center for the Disabled
Adjunct Instructor, Communication Disorders
College of Saint Rose
Albany, New York

Timothy J. Feeney, PhD
Assistant Professor, Department of Education
Project Director, Sage Neurobehavioral Resource Project
The Sage Colleges
Troy, New York

Carol M. Frattali, PhD
Research Coordinator, Speech-Language Pathology Section
W.G. Magnuson Clinical Center
National Institutes of Health
Bethesda, Maryland

Brooke Hallowell, PhD
Assistant Professor, School of Hearing and Speech Sciences
Ohio University
Athens, Ohio

Bernard P. Henri, PhD
Executive Director
Cleveland Hearing & Speech Center
Cleveland, Ohio

Alex Johnson, PhD
Director, Division of Speech-Language Sciences and Disorders, Department of Neurology
Henry Ford Hospital
Detroit, Michigan

Dorian Lee-Wilkerson, PhD
Associate Professor, Department of Communicative Sciences and Disorders
Hampton University
Hampton, Virginia

Rosemary Lubinski, EdD
Professor, Department of Communication Disorders and Sciences
University at Buffalo
Amherst, New York

Lissa Power-deFur
Associate Director, Special Education & Student Services
Virginia Department of Education
Richmond, Virginia

Nancy B. Swigert, MA
President
Swigert & Associates, Inc.
Lexington, Kentucky

Mark Ylvisaker, PhD
Associate Professor, Department of Communication Disorders
College of Saint Rose
Albany, New York

FOREWORD

PRACTICE MANAGEMENT UNDER MANAGED CARE: AN AMERICAN INVENTION, CIRCA 2000

Early in this book Becky Cornett addresses the outcomes of health care reform in the '90s and look toward the millennium for "achieving a balance between the unrestrained costs of the past and . . . restrictions placed on health care in a managed care environment." Readers will find that each chapter offers excellent on-the-cutting edge advice for speech-language pathologists in practice as well as providing practitioners-to-be insights about the sometimes incomprehensible world they are about to enter. The contributors to this text each provide a perspective that reflects upon that which has been, that which is now, and that which will be in the rapidly changing world in which those of us who have chosen this profession find ourselves.

We are not alone! Dramatic changes have occurred on many fronts. Speech-Language Pathologists have seen dramatic changes occur within all settings in which they practice. For example, there have been dramatic changes in many aspects of our scope of practice which now includes dysphagia and traumatic brain injury. Provision of appropriate services now includes the necessity to learn about more augmentative and alternative communication devices, a host of new instrumentation in medical and educational settings, an understanding of all aspects of language, going well beyond spoken language, into the arenas of reading and writing, and an understanding of linguistic and cultural diversity across the life span.

Change and its challenges are, of course, not new, although as Power-deFur points out in the closing chapter, the Information Age has made these challenges even greater. She notes that information becomes obsolete more rapidly, on the one hand, while its growth is exponential, on the other. She indicates that graduates in the year 2000 will have been exposed *in that year* to more information than their grandparents were in a lifetime.

Nevertheless, challenges have always been with us. Unfamiliarity with the contexts in which change occurs can be dangerous. This text alerts the readers to both challenges and solutions, to possible problems and probable successes. A focus on functional outcomes of assessment and treatment reflects the state-of-the-art in health care reform. With so much to learn, how is it possible to keep one's scientific, therapeutic, and professional balance? An author from an earlier era, who was greatly admired in his time, provides us with a metaphor for health care reform at the millennium.

Lewis Carroll (see Charles L. Dodgson) lived more than 100 years ago (1832–1898), but his work is still known to those who love language and are intrigued by a little girls' adventures in an unfamiliar world. Carrolls' stories illustrate well the danger and the solutions which may emerge in unsettled times. Readers know well the adventures of Alice, the protagonist. But may not recall certain passages in *Through the Looking Glass* that appear in Chapter 8, entitled "It's My Own Invention." Read on to determine who represents the gladiators of today, and who plays the role of speech language pathologist in this abridged recounting of Alice's adventures in a rapidly changing world.

Among Alice's many experiences, she awakens from a dream to find a knight in crimson armor galloping in her direction, swinging a great club and shouting that she is his prisoner. Alice was startled. However, she was also frightened for the knight, whose horse had suddenly stopped, tumbling the red knight to the ground. As he remounted his steed, another knight, known as the white knight, appeared, also falling off his steed. Having argued about who was to hold Alice as a prisoner, they finally concluded that they must fight each other, while observing regulations know as the rules of battle. Alice, hiding behind a tree, and observing the fight, could not seem to understand the rules. One of the rules that Alice had not noticed was that both knights always fell on their heads when they fell off their horses. (An example of early traumatic brain injury?) The battle ended when both fell of their respective steeds, side by side, on their heads. Then they shook hands, and the red knight galloped away.

As the white knight helped Alice on her way, Alice noted that he continued falling off his steed. As she helped him up, she mentioned that he must have had little practice in riding. He looked surprised and offended, claiming that he had plenty of practice. He concluded his protestations by saying, “The great art of riding . . . is—to keep your balance properly” (Carroll, 1865, p. 240).

There we have it! Keeping a balance between conflicting forces. Each of the several authors in this book have had considerable experience in providing desirable clinical outcomes while keeping a proper balance when faced with club-swinging forces, proving yet again, that it is possible to manage managed care. Within this text readers will find the answers to questions which arise in every day practice, and tools and techniques with which to solve dilemmas arising from the ever-changing face of health reform initiatives, which inspire new rules of battle. Carroll writes that “Of all the strange things that Alice saw on her journey *Through the Looking Glass* this was the one she always remembered most clearly. Years afterwards, she could bring the whole scene back again, as if it had been yesterday” (p. 244).

One would suspect that readers of this text will also look back from beyond the millennium to marvel at their adventures as protagonists in managed care.

Katharine G. Butler

REFERENCES

Carroll, L. 1976. The Complete Works of Lew Carroll, pp. 3–1293. New York: Random House.

PREFACE

"I just want to be a therapist. I don't want to worry about management problems." Most managers have heard their employees say this when trying to communicate with staff members about the challenges of working in health care or education settings in an era of reform. However, "managing" is not just for managers anymore. Today's speech-language pathologists work in a dynamic context in which the jobs of clinicians and managers alike depend upon shared responsibilities for knowing what work to do and how to accomplish that work in the most efficient manner. The term *clinical practice management* in the title of this book reflects the premise that each clinician is a manager of his or her own practice, and that clinical practice responsibilities include much more than the immediate patient/client-clinician relationship.

Shelly Chabon and I discussed three attitudes that are central to the clinical practice in our book *The Clinical Practice of Speech—Language Pathology* (Cornett & Chabon, 1988). We discussed three attitudes that are central to clinical practice in speech-language pathology—scientific, therapeutic, and professional. The *scientific attitude* is a commitment to evidence-based practice. Clinicians should offer services that are consistent with findings in the literature and also collect and analyze outcomes data to demonstrate the effectiveness and efficiency of their services. That is, we should know why we do what we do and be able to prove its value. The *therapeutic attitude* refers to the "heart and soul" of clinical practice—those interpersonal skills essential for creating an atmosphere in which change can occur. Most clinicians seem to focus on this attitude or set of skills as the substance of clinical practice. The *professional attitude* encompasses expertise, clinical accountability, legal and ethical behaviors, and business acumen. It is this set of skills that most clinicians would rather leave to the "managers" (except professionals in private practice, who have always been clinician-managers), who should take care of managed care issues, clinical guidelines and pathways, outcomes management, performance improvement, and other business problems.

Leading clinicians in the field have contributed to *Clinical Practice Management in Speech-Language Pathology: Principles and Practicalities*. The book is organized into three parts to help readers focus on particular aspects of clinical practice management. The chapters in Part I, "Setting the Stage: The Structure of Our Business," address managed care, outcomes measurement and management, and clinical guidelines and pathways. In Chapter 1, Bernard P. Henri and Brooke Hallowell discuss the problems and possibilities of managed care. Managed care is about managing resources—offering the right services in the right setting at the right time by the right personnel while achieving the desired outcome. Carol M. Frattali's chapter addresses outcomes management—measuring the results of care and managing treatment and other factors to achieve specific goals in the shortest period of time. The need for clinicians to demonstrate the value of speech-language pathology services in the wider context of health care and education services cannot be emphasized enough. Each clinician must be able to demonstrate that he or she is an "outcomes manager" by demonstrating that treatment makes a difference in the patient's or client's everyday life. Tracy L. Davidson and I discuss clinical guidelines, pathways, and protocols in Chapter 3. These tools help clinicians to quantify and standardize care to reduce variation in practice and to carefully plan, manage, and coordinate their efforts with other team members.

Part II presents perspectives on the functionality of assessment and treatment. Health care and educational services providers have become more familiar with the term *functional outcomes* as they have been pressed to help patients and clients achieve practical results in the shortest amount of time. A functional approach to intervention focuses on daily living skills; in this model, much more emphasis is placed on reducing disabilities (and increasing activity) and minimizing handicaps (and increasing participation in society), and much less on remediating impairments (see Chapter 2 for a full discussion of these concepts). Each of the contributors in this section is an innovator who "did" functional treatment before it was in vogue! Focusing on functional outcomes, Nancy Swigert presents a perspective on dysphagia management; Mark Ylvisaker, James Feeney, and Timothy J. Feeney address long-term rehabilitation after traumatic brain injury; Rosemary Lubinski discusses elderly patients; and Shelly S. Chabon, Dorian Lee-Wilkerson, and Noma B. Anderson reflect on sociocultural and functional perspectives. These professionals know that treatment is about making a difference in patients' everyday lives, and that the future of payment for services depends upon clinicians' ability to prove that their services result in documented value to their customers (patients/clients, family members, payers, other professionals, and the public).

To illustrate the importance of functionality—the focus on everyday-life activities—Preston Lewis wrote a scenario about the outcomes of treatment of an 18-year-old student who had participated in numerous years of "individualized instruction." Some of his comments are presented here.

- He can put 100 pegs in a board in less than 10 minutes while in his seat with 95% accuracy, but he cannot put quarters in a vending machine.
- He can sing the alphabet and recite the names of the letters when presented on a card with 80% accuracy, but he is unable to distinguish the men's room from the ladies' room at McDonald's.
- He can sort blocks by color, up to 10 different colors, but he cannot sort white from dark clothes for the washing machine.
- He can identify with 100% accuracy 100 different Peabody picture cards by pointing, but he is unable to order a hamburger by pointing to a picture on a menu or by gesturing.
- He can count to 100 by rote memory, but he does not know how many dollars to pay the clerk for a $2.59 McDonald's coupon special.

Part III of this book, which examines the future of speech-language pathology, is both fun and challenging. The fun part is having free rein to present ideas, dreams, and musings about the future of the profession; the hard part is speculating on what might be a cloudy future as health care and educational reforms continue. Focusing on the future of the profession, Alex Johnson examines health care settings, and Lissa Power-deFur discusses education settings.

Many persons have contributed to the concepts, format, writing, and production of this book. I am particularly indebted to the contributors, without whom there would be no book. Many thanks also to Sandy Cannon, Acquisitions Editor, and Mary Anne Langdon, Developmental Editor, at Aspen Publishers, Inc.; Dr. Kay Butler for her guidance and expertise; Debbie Kravitz at The Ohio State University Medical Center for her assistance in preparing the manuscript; Dr. Shelly Chabon, Dr. Herb Rubin, and Karen Seelig—my mentors in the field of speech-language pathology; my colleague and friend, Dr. Carol Frattali, who continues to inspire my work; and my family, Skip and Andrea Cornett, for their support.

I hope that the outcome of this book is greater understanding, increased skills, and renewed commitment to clinical practice, to the speech-language pathology profession, and to individuals with communication disorders and their families.

REFERENCES

Cornett, B. & Chabon, S. (1988). The clinical practice of speech-language pathology. Columbus, OH: Merrill.

PART I

Setting the Stage: The Structure of Our Business

The last decade has been an era of health care reform as high health care costs have been questioned and managed care systems established to contain these costs. The next decade promises to be an era of managed care reform, as we attempt to achieve a balance between the unrestrained costs of the past and allegations of too many restrictions placed on health care in the managed care environment. According to the Center for Health Professions at the University of California, San Francisco (1998, pp. 1, 4), successful practitioners will be those who do the following:

- Think systemically, rather than on an individual patient basis.
- Adopt management skills.
- Collaborate with others.
- Seek insight from professionals outside the health care industry.
- Constantly adapt to the market.

The three chapters in this section provide context for conducting the business of speech-language pathology—evaluating and treating persons with communication and related disorders. The contributors help clinicians to understand the fiscal environment, to focus on measuring and managing outcomes, and to incorporate clinical decision-making tools into their practice to achieve results. These chapters facilitate clinicians' understanding of managed care's core mission—"to deliver just the right care, in the right setting, using just the right resources, all in an effort to yield desirable clinical outcomes in the most cost-effective manner" (Harvey & DePue, 1997, p. 39).

An excellent illustration of the goal of Part I is a scenario presented in the *ASHA Leader* titled "Using Advocacy in Health Care Settings" (Davolt, 1998). A hospital-based speech-language pathologist learned that hemiparetic stroke patients were not being referred routinely for speech-language pathology evaluations. She conducted an extensive review of the literature and gave a presentation to the hospital's neurologists and a hospital oversight committee on the value of speech-language pathology services for this population. As a result of the evidence she presented, speech-language pathology services were added to the hospital's clinical pathway for stroke patients on a trial basis for one year. After the first year, the services were included permanently. This speech-language pathologist was able to be a successful advocate and business manager, based upon her ability to apply clinical practice management principles to a demanding situation in her workplace.

REFERENCES

Center for the Health Professions at the University of California, San Francisco (1998). Changing health care system demands new leaders. *Front & Center, 2* (3), 1–5.

Davolt, S. (1998, October 20). Using advocacy in health care settings. *ASHA Leader, 3* (20), 1, 6.

Harvey, N., & DePue, D. (1997, June). Disease management: A continuum approach. *Healthcare Financial Management*, 38–42.

CHAPTER 1

Mastering Managed Care: Problems and Possibilities

Bernard P. Henri and Brooke Hallowell

Objectives

- Describe the goals of managed care.
- Identify key challenges to the practice of speech-language pathology and audiology in the managed care marketplace.
- Describe the changing roles of speech-language pathologists in today's health care system.
- Identify the four medical-necessity criteria for clinical services.
- Develop legislative, regulatory, and private-sector advocacy strategies for speech-language pathology services.

INTRODUCTION

The service delivery trends and health care financing philosophy inspired by the managed care industry are having a profound and rapidly expanding impact on the professions of speech-language pathology and audiology, and on persons with communication and swallowing disorders. This chapter reviews the goals of managed care; discusses current trends, some with positive and some with negative implications for clinical practice; and presents several specific ways in which alterations in clinical practice may help to meet the myriad challenges associated with new modes of service delivery.

DEFINITIONS AND GOALS OF MANAGED CARE

There are numerous definitions of managed care in the health care literature. Some focus on its aims of maximizing health outcomes, preventing illness, coordinating care, and reducing unnecessary care. Others (Griffin & Fazen, 1993) focus on specific cost-control and cost-cutting tactics that are characteristic of managed care service delivery, such as those described in the following pages. The three most frequently stated goals of managed care are assurance of the quality and coordination of care, access to care for persons who need it, and cost control.

THE PERVASIVENESS OF MANAGED CARE

The rapid proliferation of managed care practices in the United States has had a dramatic influence on virtually all aspects of service delivery to persons with communication and swallowing disorders. Estimates pertaining to managed care market penetration in the United States are highly variable, because of (1) tremendous variability in managed care proliferation according to geographic location and (2) variability in the definition of what constitutes "managed care." The Health Care Financing Administration (HCFA) reports that 32% of Medicaid enrollees received benefits through managed care contracts in 1996, and that number continues to rise steadily. Of enrollees in employer-sponsored health care plans in 1997, 71% received their health care services through a managed care arrangement (Oberlander, 1997).

However, these percentages may be misleading. Today, cost-control mechanisms are practiced not only within managed care organizations (MCOs) but also in traditional fee-for-service insurance arrangements and as part of the federally sponsored Medicare and Medicaid health care programs. These mechanisms include increasingly stringent utilization review; preadmission certification for hospital stays; required preauthorization for services; negotiated reduced reimbursement rates; designation of a restricted list of preferred providers; the designation of physicians as "gatekeepers" of patients' access to health care services; salaried employment of physicians by payer organizations; incentives for physicians not to refer patients to specialty services (such as rehabilitation services); use of red-flag diagnostic or treatment categories to deny reimbursement; and restrictions on frequency, intensity, and duration of care. Therefore, the actual penetration rate of managed care across the country is now close to 100% (Hallowell & Henri, 1997).

The health care industry will certainly continue to evolve, as providers and consumers advocate for reforms, new regulations are developed to cope with some of the problems associated with managed care, and corporate health care providers face increasing competition (Swartz & Brennan, 1996). But regardless of the specific details of its evolution, and regardless of professional contexts, speech-language pathologists and audiologists will continue to provide most of their services in speech-language pathology and audiology through avenues that are heavily influenced by managed care.

WHY BE CONCERNED ABOUT MANAGED CARE?

Although the three main goals of managed care—quality and coordination of care, access to care, and cost control—are desirable, recent developments suggest that managed care is not conducive to progress in terms of quality of care or access to health care (Engelhard & Childress, 1995; Henri & Hallowell, 1996; Smith & Ashbaugh, 1995). This is because cost control is receiving much greater emphasis than quality of care and access to care. In addition, many of the initial savings projected by managed care policy makers are being outweighed by the increasing costs associated with the corporatization of health care and, ironically, the administration of cost-saving schemes (Hillman, 1995).

Consumers' and health care providers' increasing frustrations with the constraints and bureaucratic obstacles of managed care are frequently highlighted in the news media and the popular press, reflecting the reality that the American public is becoming dissatisfied with the effects of managed care on health care service delivery. Public trust in the health care system is at stake largely because of the erosion of consumers' trust that health care providers will respect the needs of the patient over economic considerations (Mechanic, 1996).

Managed care trends present numerous concerns that are particularly pertinent to the professions of speech-language pathology and audiology. The key challenges can be placed into five broad categories: (1) consumers' access to services; (2) the quality, intensity, duration, and frequency of care that is provided; (3) the fiscal stability of service-providing agencies; (4) the livelihood of professionals in the field; and (5) the maintenance of professional integrity. Each of these challenges is briefly discussed below.

Problems of Consumers' Access to Services

Consumers' access to diagnostic and treatment services under managed care is threatened by decreased referrals from gatekeepers—usually physicians, who often receive financial incentives to decrease the number of services offered to patients. Particularly problematic for some subpopulations who are in particular need of speech-language pathology services is managed care's focus on acute care. Within this model of service delivery, a principal way in which clinicians are held accountable for the outcomes of their services is through the documentation of patients' consistent improvements throughout a treatment program, leading up to an optimal point of discharge based on maximal progress. Consequently, persons with chronic disability, multiple disabilities, or degenerative conditions (Fox, Wicks, & Newacheck, 1993; Smith & Ashbaugh, 1995) and persons who are elderly (Clement, Retchin, Brown, & Stegall, 1994; Oberlander, 1997) are finding it more and more difficult to receive speech-language pathology services. Furthermore, such persons are less likely to receive full insurance coverage by MCOs (Iglehart, 1995), primarily because of preexisting condition clauses (restrictions based on conditions diagnosed prior to the enrollment). MCOs appear to be far more selective in their enrollments than were the traditional indemnity insurance carriers, with MCOs avoiding coverage of individuals whose care will be more costly (Clement et al., 1994; Fisher, 1994; Perkins, 1998).

Additional subpopulations with restricted access to care include low-income populations and members of cultural and ethnic minorities (Henri & Hallowell, 1996; Leigh, 1994; Stenger, 1993). Although the research literature lacks empirical backing for the causes posited for this restricted or discriminatory access, some possible reasons are that members of these subpopulations are less likely to enjoy employer-sponsored health care plans, are less likely to be able to afford their own health care coverage, and may be less likely to advocate for their own health care coverage needs (Purtilo, 1995). Unfortunately, members of these subpopulations have a disproportionately greater need for speech-language pathology rehabilitation services (Hillman, 1995; Screen & Anderson, 1994).

Another barrier to care is the tendency on the part of MCOs to "lock out" nonphysician providers, by contending that there is adequate representation of specialties in the provider panels to cover enrollees' needs, even though certain types of specialties (such as speech-language pathology and/or audiology) are not represented. By stating that all services provided must meet specific criteria for medical necessity (Moore & Rabins, 1996), MCOs exercise a more subtle form of lockout. MCOs argue that most of the services provided by speech-language pathologists and audiologists fall outside the rubric of medical necessity. A new concept threatening to worsen the lockout of these disciplines from the ranks of covered service providers is the concept of "evidence-based" medical necessity, wherein payers require evidence of a solid body of well-controlled research to support the effectiveness of any intervention administered ("Medicare HMOs," 1998). This requirement will present new challenges to all care providers.

Concerns about Quality, Intensity, Duration, and Frequency of Care

Restrictions on duration and frequency of treatments (Gill, 1995) are a hallmark cost-containment feature of managed care plans that affect speech-language pathologists' ability to offer all of the services that might benefit clients. Some MCOs simply restrict the number of treatment sessions an enrollee may receive in a given period of time following the onset of a particular diagnosis (such as 10 or 20 sessions of speech-language treatment after a patient suffers a cerebrovascular accident). Others limit services to a specific range of professionals (such as allowing 20 visits for speech-language pathology, physical therapy, and occupational therapy services, combined). Such restrictions frequently limit professionals' abilities to bring about significant functional progress, despite the promising rehabilitation potential of the individuals they serve. These restrictions also create the possibility of a circular process; when little progress is made because few visits are permitted, the insurer denies further care because little progress was made.

Perhaps the most salient factor affecting the quality of speech-language pathology services is the increased intervention of insurance companies in matters that traditionally have been the responsibility of clinicians (such as planning treatment; setting goals; determining frequency and duration of services; specifying treatment approaches; determining adequate progress; and selecting which products or equipment the patient needs). In addition, interruptions in the continuity of care occur more often due to delays in authorization and reauthorization for services. Although the use of assistants and aides in the treatment of communication and swallowing disorders is relatively new, there are growing concerns that the overuse and misuse of these less-expensive (and less-qualified) personnel may result in further reductions in the quality and outcomes of care.

Ironically, as monitoring the quality of care has gained increased attention under managed care, MCOs have tended to minimize quality improvement practices in efforts to further reduce their own costs (Fisher, 1994). Recent research examining quality of health care suggests that reliance upon accreditation mechanisms, such as the National Committee on Quality Assurance (NCQA), can be deceptive, especially because high percentages of MCOs' dissatisfied enrollees withdraw from membership and thus are not included in consumer satisfaction or other quality surveys ("Medicare HMOs," 1998).

Concerns about the Fiscal Stability of Service-Providing Agencies

Because MCOs negotiate lower fees for services with the providers with whom they establish service contracts, payments for speech-language pathologists' services under managed care are decreasing, with reported discounts ranging from 20% to 80%. Moreover, processing time for claims by insurance carriers is increasing. At one time, payment for services was received in as few as 15 days from the billing date, but now may take several months and, in some instances, over a year. Dramatic increases in the frequency of claims denials for services rendered further threaten the fiscal stability of service providers. At the same time, administrative and bureaucratic obstacles are being added, which increase administrative costs. Agencies that provide services are adjusting their operations accordingly, by reducing numbers of employees, competing with other agencies for additional service contracts, expanding marketing efforts, and enforcing rigorous clinical productivity standards.

Concerns about the Livelihood of Speech-Language Pathologists

As service providers address fiscal challenges, some effects on the availability of jobs and on salary levels are inevitable. Many speech-language pathology professionals have personally experienced the effects of reengineering, consolidation, and downsizing movements in hospitals, community speech and hearing centers, private practice agencies, and rehabilitation companies. Fortunately, the continuous growth of populations requiring the skilled services of speech-language pathologists—including elderly persons, persons surviving traumatic injuries and life-threatening illness, and children with multiple handicaps—helps to offset the impact of managed care on employment prospects for clinicians.

Concerns about Maintaining Professional Integrity

Two parallel trends in service delivery under managed care pose some threat to the integrity of the professions of speech-language pathology and audiology as we know them. One involves increased use of assistants, technicians, and aides in areas of clinical practice that were once exclusively in the domain of licensed and/or certified clinicians (American Speech-Language-Hearing Association, 1996a; Gerard, 1990; Holzemer, 1996). The other trend involves the increased emphasis on multiskilling, or transdisciplinary training of health care professionals, which may lessen the specialized expertise of some professionals offering services. As a result of these trends, the level of skill, education, training, licensure, certification, and overall competence of clinical practitioners is likely to become less consistent across various treatment settings. Although there are merits to some of the arguments for the use of support and/or cross-trained personnel in some environments, it is very important that today's clinicians take seriously their roles as advocates for their profession's integrity.

THE GOOD NEWS

Although practitioners generally agree that managed care's consequences are far more negative than positive, its positive consequences are important to recognize, too. The emphasis on preventive care and health maintenance and the reduced health care costs for many covered individuals are benefits that virtually all MCOs tout and that most managed care enrollees enjoy. Perhaps the most important positive impact of managed care on speech-language pathology and audiology is the increased accountability of clinicians and service-providing agencies.

More than ever before, providers of clinical services are required to ensure that services provided are necessary, and that those services address important life-affecting changes in clients and patients. Once trained to think of treatment in terms of clinical, performance-based objectives (for example, objectives pertaining to grammatical rules, articulator placement, or speech sound discrimination—remote from practical communication in real-world contexts), clinicians have been challenged to reformulate diagnostic and treatment activities to take into account functional outcomes.

An additional positive impact of managed care related to the increased focus on professional accountability is the increased documentation of and research on treatment efficacy and treatment outcomes (American Speech-Language-Hearing Association, Task Force on Treatment Outcomes and Cost Effectiveness, 1995, 1997). The fact that third-party payers and government-sponsored health care plans are now requiring data about these aspects of services in order to justify paying for them has stimulated professional organizations, researchers, and clinicians to generate such data. Although there continues to be a paucity of controlled, clinical research in speech-language pathology and audiology, some university research and teaching programs have reorganized research and teaching priorities during the past 10 years so that clinical research is encouraged much more than before (Minifie, 1997). Likewise, federal, state, and private funding opportunities for research involving treatment outcomes and treatment efficacy have been on the rise. The trend toward more controlled research regarding clinical practices will undoubtedly help clinicians not only justify their services but also learn better ways to diagnose, treat, and make valid prognostic statements about a wide range of communication and swallowing disorders.

The National Center for Treatment Effectiveness in Communication Disorders (NCTECD), a new program of the American Speech-Language-Hearing Association (ASHA), has been established to coordinate all outcomes and efficacy work for the Association (NCTECD, 1999). NCTECD is developing and implementing the National Outcomes Measurement System (NOMS) to assist practitioners working with adults and children in educational and health care environments. ASHA hopes that the use of NOMS will provide speech-language pathologists and audiologists with the tools they need to advocate at the state and federal level for their services, convince payers and administrators of the value of their services, change practice patterns, and improve the quality of services (NCTECD,

1999). The database underpinning NOMS will be developed using the Functional Communication Measures, a seven-point scale scored by speech-language pathologists at admission and discharge. Changes in scores will help to determine the effectiveness of treatment.

In addition, managed care has made speech-language pathologists and audiologists increasingly aware of the financial impact of their individual and agencywide services on the financial well-being of their employing agencies. Although clinicians once expected to perform their clinical duties without monitoring clinical revenues, clinicians now frequently play a vital role in the business and financial planning teamwork within their agencies. Many clinical professionals report that this change has increased their sense of ownership for their agency's operations. Likewise, employers report improved business savvy of their clinical employees (Henri & Hallowell, 1997b).

As new formulas for practice under changing modes of service delivery continue to evolve, it is likely that speech-language pathologists and audiologists will continue to see further positive effects on their professions—such as more efficient and increasingly outcome-focused treatments; new types of employment opportunities (such as opportunities for aides and assistants); and improved interdisciplinary teamwork in coordination of patient care, cotreatment, and discharge planning. The active role that speech-language pathologists and audiologists play as advocates for their clients and for their professions is critical to maximizing the positive aspects of managed care.

NECESSARY PRACTICE ADJUSTMENTS IN AN ERA OF CHANGE

The Changing Role of the Speech-Language Pathologist

Speech-language pathologists, regardless of practice setting, must adjust their client and patient interactions to correspond to this new health care financing environment. Clinicians who fail to recognize the necessity of adjusting their practice patterns will find themselves excluded from the practice panels of MCOs.

Paradoxically, although insurance companies are driving the changing role of speech-language pathologists, they are not yet adjusting their payment policies and practices to be consistent with these role adjustments. MCOs and health maintenance organizations (HMOs) continue to pay primarily for traditional services (that is, one-on-one treatment provided by a licensed, fully credentialed practitioner) by way of discounted fee-for-service schedules. The low incidence of communication and swallowing disorders in the general population and the resulting low utilization of speech-language pathologists' services continue to make capitated payment (a predetermined, negotiated monthly payment per enrollee paid to a provider) and prospective payment (predetermined based on diagnosis) costly payment methods for fixed payment payers and providers to administer. Some providers of speech-language pathology services, however, are engaged in capitated and subcapitated service contracts.

Gill (1995) rather bluntly describes the changes occurring in ambulatory rehabilitation care delivery:

> Because decreasing expenses are key in the capitated environment, . . . most treatment sessions are between 30 and 45 minutes, length of treatment is closer to 6 visits per admission, nonprofessional support personnel and group sessions are widely used, and significant attention is paid to patient education and home programming. Investments are made in support staff education and the supervisory training of therapists. Such staff development efforts are critical to the capitated environment as low cost resources are required for efficient care delivery. Licensed therapists are trained to plan and evaluate treatment and to supervise the treatment provided by nonlicensed staff. . . .
>
> For this model to be successful, therapists must assume the evaluator/supervisor role, in which they evaluate the patient and develop the plan of care. During treatment, their role is to reevaluate and update the plan while others provide the hands-on care. Although most therapists are not in favor of this model of care, the one-to-one treatment model can no longer be an affordable option. And until therapists can prove that other models are less effective, payors will not listen. (p. SC–14)

Clearly, as managed care evolves, a necessary consequence will be a significant change in the traditional role of the speech-language pathologist. The one-on-one, long-term treatment arrangements of the past will continue to decline in both health care and educational settings. Although common not too long ago, treatment durations of 12 to 18 months for persons with cerebrovascular accidents, degenerative nervous system diseases, or traumatic brain injuries are already vanishing and being replaced with far shorter periods (such as 60 days). Reduced access and greatly restricted visits will compel speech-language pathologists to adopt the roles of diagnostician, treatment planner, and supervisor. As clients' care is carried out by trained family caregivers or support staff and multiskilled personnel, the speech-language pathologist will be engaged increasingly in the role of consultant—reviewing and modifying treatment plans and demonstrating techniques to instruct the care extenders about the most effective interventions. In summary, a likely scenario is that the fully credentialed speech-language pathologist will function as diagnostician, treatment planner, and supervisor, guiding the entire process of care from admission to discharge.

Clinical Productivity

As revenues for services continue to drop (in some instances by as much as 20% to 25%) and as employers strive to maintain fiscal stability while providing competitive compensation packages and state-of-the-art facilities and instrumentation, clinical productivity requirements are increasing. Whereas in 1989, clinicians delivered an average of 23.9 weekly hours of client/patient contact (American Speech-Language-Hearing Association, Strategic Resources Group, 1991), clinicians today are required to deliver an average of 30 to 32 hours per week of care, or 6 to 6.5 hours of patient contact per day. Some clinicians report required productivity levels of 37.5 hours weekly (Hallowell & Henri, 1997). Increasingly, speech-language pathologists are being required to provide group therapy to generate required hourly revenues and to protect against the financial consequences of appointment cancellations. Missed or canceled appointments, which are today being far more vigorously addressed, are being re-scheduled as quickly as possible. To ensure that clinicians attain the necessary contact hours or clinical encounters of service to balance budgets, organizations are requiring flexible weekly work schedules and evening and weekend hours.

In addition, many agencies are adopting financial and nonfinancial, productivity-based incentive systems to maximize units delivered per clinician, thus keeping personnel and related expenses under control. Although incentive systems are only beginning to appear in not-for-profit environments, they have been used for several years in for-profit rehabilitation service settings. Such systems may be effective in increasing clinical revenues, but it is essential that they are designed and implemented carefully to lessen possible ethical, administrative, and financial pitfalls (Henri & Hallowell, 1997a).

To ensure the referrals needed to sustain productivity goals for speech-language pathology programs, organizations are developing comprehensive marketing programs with components emphasizing the impact of these services upon quality of life, reduced burdens on caregivers, and improved medical management of patients (Hoen, Thelander, & Worsely, 1997; Mason, 1996; Records, Tomblin, & Freese, 1992; Smith et al., 1996). As an additional avenue for obtaining referrals and improving the financial return on marketing investments and efforts, organizations are forming alliances with other organizations to offer a broader spectrum of services (Hallowell, Henri, & Napp, 1997). For example, providers offering speech-language pathology and audiology services are developing joint ventures with entities offering physical and occupational therapy and social work services. These systems are developing collaborative and coordinated marketing plans to ensure that resources are being used to obtain maximum impact and results.

Adjustments in Hiring and Staffing

The rapidly changing health care environment requires clinicians to be far more flexible and adaptable in their work attitude and outlook. To prosper within managed care environments, speech-language pathologists must be entrepreneurial, willing to learn more about the financial and business aspects of clinical practice (Goldberg, 1996). To ensure the fiscal stability of their organizations and their own livelihood, clinicians practicing in the managed care environment must be active participants in their employers' marketing strategies and activities (Ashby, 1995). They must also become skilled contract negotiators (Breakey, 1994; Vekovius, 1995).

For clinicians to remain competitive, it is essential that they have a commitment to life-long learning to enhance their clinical skills and also their interpersonal and business skills (Vekovius, 1995). The decreased length of stay and number of allowed visits, along with escalating productivity demands, are creating pressures to maintain state-of-the-art knowledge concerning the most cost-effective management of communication and swallowing disorders. Only speech-language pathologists with a solid and current knowledge base will be able to deliver the most effective, quality care. Clinicians must keep abreast of the applied clinical research literature. Various strategies to support continued learning—such as participating in continuing education and distance learning activities, grand rounds, and monthly study groups—must be implemented.

Speech-language pathologists who fall behind in their knowledge base may soon find themselves eased out of provider panels due to inefficiencies in clinical practice or less favorable clinical outcomes than those of other practitioners. Or, employers will compel these individuals to upgrade their skills to maintain employment. Examples of cutting edge clinical procedures requiring ongoing training of clinicians now in the workplace are intraoperative monitoring (Hall, 1992) and fiberoptic endoscopic examination of swallowing (FEES) (Kidder, Langmore, & Martin, 1994).

Employers will seek individuals who have multiple skills as one way of reducing costs (Pietranton & Lynch, 1995). Employers will vigorously pursue persons who are computer literate and able to navigate the Internet to acquire information necessary to provide the most cost-effective care possible. Because teams are now vital in most service delivery contexts, process skills such as leadership, transdisciplinary teamwork, and interdisciplinary communication are critical (Goldberg, 1996).

Speech-language pathologists must become more assertive advocates on behalf of their clients (Hallowell & Henri, 1997, 1998). Because clinicians have a greater understanding of the complexities associated with managed care, it is incumbent upon them to participate in the education of their consumers. Practitioners must also educate primary care physicians, MCO/HMO officials, legislators, and other individuals able to effect positive changes in policies and practices that undermine clinicians' capacity to serve. Efforts to overturn authorization and treatment denials are now the combined responsibility of speech-language pathologists and consumers, often assisted by physicians.

Alternative Treatment Approaches

With resources rapidly diminishing, it is necessary to explore alternative ways of providing speech-language pathology services. For some practitioners who have worked in poverty-stricken or rural parts of the country where resources have always been at a premium, little may change. For years, these clinicians have been compelled to develop creative solutions to address inadequate resources for treatment. Much can be learned from these individuals. Now all practitioners, regardless of setting, are having to explore ways of maximizing treatment resources. Today, the principle of "do more with less" is fully operational. As a result, alternative approaches to delivering services must be developed.

Increased Use of Support Personnel

The use of support personnel remains particularly controversial in the field of speech-language pathology. Clinicians who support this idea believe it to be an effective method to relieve the challenges of providing effective services to large caseloads, to match the level of care needed with level of training and experience, and to allow more time for the treatment of individuals with severe and complex communication disorders; thus proponents argue that the use of support personnel will improve the overall quality of care. Opponents fear that the quality of patient care will be diminished and that their job security will be eroded. Some are concerned that cost-minded health care and educational administrators will compel assistants to provide services outside their prescribed scope of practice and implement practices that exceed appropriate supervisor-to-support staff ratios.

An additional and substantial problem is that many MCOs/HMOs still do not recognize support personnel as qualified providers of speech-language pathology services and therefore do not pay for treatment delivered by these persons. Nevertheless, in some contexts, speech-language pathology assistants and aides can help to obtain optimal treatment results by supplementing and supporting treatment designed by speech-language pathologists. Activities can include performing articulation drills, conducting oral motor exercises, and monitoring computer-assisted treatment (Kimbarow, 1997). Support staff can also contribute to the efficiency of fully qualified clinicians by helping to prepare treatment and caregiver materials, transporting patients to treatment in patient settings, and recordkeeping.

Multiskilled Professionals

"Multiskilling" is another controversial strategy to increase the effectiveness, efficiency, and coordination of health care services delivery

(Pietranton & Lynch, 1995). The multiskilled professional is one who has been cross-trained to perform functions that formerly were the sole responsibility of another professional (American Speech-Language-Hearing Association, 1997c). However, as Pietranton and Lynch (1995) emphasize, there remains much uncertainty about the responsibilities and required skills of multiskilled professionals.

Graduate Externs

Graduate externs have served as a readily-available source of trained personnel for the provision of properly-supervised evaluation and treatment services. Patients and clients, who understand the need to prepare future practitioners, have traditionally accepted the use of graduate students. Many patients, in fact, are pleased that they can participate in externs' training. However, the effects of MCO/HMO credentialing requirements upon the continued availability of these individuals to deliver services is unclear.

Trained Volunteers

Another treatment extender is the trained volunteer. Periodically, individuals with backgrounds in helping professions want to work in some way with clients. Because no compensation is involved, and because these individuals are clearly identified to clients as volunteers, there are fewer legal and no licensure-related problems. Their purpose is presented as that of providing, at no financial cost to the client, additional opportunities to practice and maintain developing skills in the presence of another person (Lyon, 1992). Before they provide direct patient services, volunteers may be required to observe treatment sessions; then they may be guided by the speech-language pathologist in the provision of limited treatment-reinforcing activities such as repetitive drills.

Family Members and Other Caregivers

As managed care continues to expand, family members are often required to provide health care services to their loved ones. As with trained volunteers, coaching and training by the speech-language pathologist is essential. It has long been recognized that treatment-complementing activities provided by a properly guided caregiver can be highly effective (Des Rosier, Cantanzaro, & Piller, 1992; Evans, Bishop, & Haselkorn, 1991). With increased family member involvement, it will become necessary to identify the unique variables that minimize or prevent successful caregiver follow-through at home or elsewhere (Scott, 1998).

The trend toward increased caregiver involvement constitutes one of the unacknowledged, hidden costs of the shift in who is really paying for care. Family members are having to take time off from work to manage or deliver a parent's, spouse's, partner's, or child's rehabilitation services. Today, caregivers provide up to three hours per day of guided treatment, and they now feel the responsibility for treatment outcomes (M. Burnett, personal communication, August 5, 1998). Employers are beginning to experience the reduced productivity and therefore costly consequences of a partially disengaged workforce conflicted between the demanding obligations of home and work. Although employers have decreased their primary health care expenditures, the costs of these hidden "health care" expenses have yet to be computed. The impact of legislation such as the Family and Medical Leave Act has not yet been determined.

Increased Efficiency and Effectiveness

Today's managed care philosophy is propelling changes in the duration and content of speech-language pathology evaluation and treatment services. It is now necessary to increase the efficiency and effectiveness of the manner in which evaluations, treatment, and report writing occur. Accurate diagnoses of speech-language disorders will have to be derived more quickly. Caregiver training must occur during the limited treatment visits allowed by MCOs/HMOs, so that services can be extended and results improved without increasing costs.

Changes in Documentation

Documentation of evaluation and treatment services is also being affected by managed care. Although the lengthy evaluation report produced in graduate school may be useful as a pedagogical tool, it is not appropriate in the managed care environment because it is too expensive to create, produce, distribute, and store. Clinicians today must generate reports that are brief (some limited to small portions of preprinted forms, others allowing one to two pages) and yet provide the information required by referral sources and payers. Typically, these requirements include a brief statement of history and presenting problem; results, in summary form, of formal and informal assessment; outcome-oriented, long-range goals; the diagnosis and prognosis; and, if possible, the estimated duration of treatment. Most payers require periodic, brief progress reports that describe progress toward the initial goals and objectives. Any modifications of goals must be specified and justified. Notes must correspond to each treatment session. Generally, the content of these notes must address the degree of progress made toward the goals and objectives. Should a daily encounter be undocumented, utilization reviewers may require that reimbursement be refunded (Henri & Cornett, 1992). A specific challenge facing speech-language pathologists and audiologists (and all other practitioners) is the need to document clinical outcomes and treatment costs through accurate, comparative data (American Speech-Language-Hearing Association, Task Force on Treatment Outcomes, 1995).

Medical Necessity

One of the most frequent reasons cited by insurers in their denial of service, whether for treatment authorization or payments, is that the care delivered is not "medically necessary." To meet narrow medical-necessity standards, the condition being treated must sometimes proceed directly from an illness or injury. Kahan et al. (1994, pp. 357–359) provide helpful direction in supporting the medical necessity of clinical services. They present the following four criteria:

1. The procedure must be appropriate (that is, its benefits must sufficiently outweigh its risks to make it worth performing, and it must do at least as well as the next-best available procedure).
2. It would be improper care not to recommend this service.
3. There is reasonable chance that the procedure will benefit the patient.
4. The benefit to the patient is not small.

Perkins and Olson (1998) provide further guidance to support the medical necessity of speech-language pathology services. Their definition states that medically necessary care is the care that, in the opinion of the treating physician, is reasonably needed to accomplish one or more of the following:

- to prevent the onset or worsening of an illness, condition, or disability
- to establish a diagnosis
- to provide palliative, curative, or restorative treatment for physical and/or mental health conditions
- to assist the individual to achieve or maintain maximum functional capacity in performing daily activities, taking into account both the functional capacity of the individual and those functional capacities that are appropriate for individuals of the same age

Perkins and Olson (1997) further argue that each service must be sufficient in amount, duration, and scope to reasonably achieve its purpose; and the amount, duration, and scope may not arbitrarily be denied or reduced solely because of the diagnosis, type of illness, or condition.

Evidence-based medical necessity is another method recently used by insurers to decrease health care costs by decreasing the number of authorizations and payment amounts. Insurance companies are required, by federal law, to pay only for those treatments having demonstrated effectiveness. Thus, some MCOs/HMOs reimburse only for services where controlled research supports the effectiveness of a particular intervention (Frattali, 1990–91; "The Threat of Evidence-Based Definitions," 1998).

The frequent use of strict medical-necessity standards as a means of denying care reinforces the mandate that speech-language pathologists and audiologists must maintain an up-to-date command of their research and treatment literature and have access to and use all available reference materials to support their management of communication and swallowing disorders.

The Need for Functional Treatment Outcomes

In all instances, care provided to persons with communication and swallowing disorders must be measured against its impact upon functional outcomes—that is, its impact upon the patient's daily quality of life. This is the stated priority with all MCOs/HMOs. Insurers also want to know with greater definitiveness what the outcomes of treatment will be versus the costs invested. Speech-language pathologists and audiologists must be able to document patient/client outcomes and costs for treatment through accurate, comparative data (Keatley, Miller, & Mann, 1995).

The Role of Technology in Managed Care

It is necessary today to identify the specific areas where technology can be used reliably and cost-effectively to minimize the costs of speech-language intervention and to improve clinical outcomes (American Speech-Language-Hearing Association, 1997d). Computer-assisted evaluation and treatment are becoming more available in most clinical environments. Software that accelerates the process of language and phonology systems analysis has long been in existence. Reports, referral acknowledgments, and collection letters can all be generated from templates contained in word-processing packages. The outcomes and costs of treatment can be monitored using computer-based software (Keatley et al., 1995).

The Internet now makes it possible for clinicians and consumers to access experts ("hyperspecialists") anywhere in the world to obtain consultation and guidance concerning the management of difficult, complex, or rare cases. Evaluation and treatment no longer have to be confined to the hospital treatment room or other health care or educational settings. "Distance treatment" is technologically possible today, via the Internet (Goldberg, 1996) and interactive video (Goldberg, 1997). The cost-reduction pressures of managed care dictate that all of these technologically based avenues be explored and adopted, when appropriate.

Although technology can be very attractive, the use of expensive instrumentation can lead to increased costs in service delivery. Providers must consider the lifespan of equipment, the reimbursability of procedures using instrumentation, and the maintenance costs when contemplating the purchase of expensive devices. Certainly, the costs of acquiring any technology must be weighed carefully against the benefits to be obtained in terms of reducing the cost of delivering care and improving treatment outcomes (Hallowell & Katz, in press).

Ethical Considerations

Speech-language pathologists providing services in managed care's arena of diminishing resources are ethically obligated to ensure that increasingly scarce health care resources are being used as effectively as possible, that the clinical return on resource investment is reasonable (O'Malley, 1997). More than ever, speech-language pathologists and audiologists, pressured by demands for maximum clinical productivity, find themselves torn between quality of patient care considerations and the pressures to reduce costs. Often, their fiduciary responsibilities (keeping the interests of their patients foremost) are in direct conflict with the financial responsibilities dictated to them by the MCOs/HMOs (Callahan, 1992). Incentives—whether to provide or not to provide care—create the possibility for additional ethical conflict and stress (Henri & Hallowell, 1997a).

The American Speech-Language-Hearing Association's "Code of Ethics" (1994) and *Preferred Practice Patterns* (1997a, 1997b) provide a useful foundation to guide speech-language pathologists in addressing ethical dilemmas (Hallowell & Henri, 1997, 1998). Further guidance can be derived from use of clinical pathways (Cornett, 1994), which are standard procedures for assessment, treatment, and management based on diagnosis or disorder (see Chapter 3). Speech-language pathologists have had an opportunity for substantial input in the development of pathways and clinical guidelines in health care organizations.

Actions for Advocacy

To ensure patient/client access to speech-language pathology services, agencies that provide these services must address the growing number of payment denials by insurers. The denial rates for evaluations and treatment authorizations at some agencies have grown by as much as six times the level of two years ago, going from 5% to 30% (Hallowell & Henri, 1998). Because it is far less expensive to prevent than appeal denials, a helpful strategy has been for agencies to identify the four or five MCOs/HMOs funding the largest percentage of their patients' services. Once these insurers/payers have been identified, the agency's provider relations departments should learn the specific requirements concerning documentation, authorization, billing, payment, and appeal of denials. This information should be maintained in writing within the appropriate department(s) of the agency.

Should denials occur despite these preventive measures, there is greater than a 90% chance that they can be overturned (Hallowell & Henri, 1998).

Therefore, 100% of denials should be appealed. Typically, what is needed is a written request for authorization by the primary care physician or additional, supporting documentation resulting from the evaluation or treatment. Another productive tactic is having the patient file a complaint with his or her employer's human resources department, with a copy sent to the insurer. Finally, a more confrontational measure is to inform the MCO/HMO that a complaint will be filed with the state's insurance commissioner. It is important to maintain a cooperative rather than adversarial attitude throughout the process of denial reversal to avoid undermining relationships with the insurer.

Although advocacy by consumers themselves is usually very effective, consumers who have communication disorders are less likely to advocate for the services they or their family members need. In these situations, it is the responsibility of the clinician to provide the consumer with the information necessary to be an effective self-advocate. Guidance can be provided concerning how to approach primary care physicians and insurers, to reverse prior authorization or treatment denials, to write letters to legislators and insurance commissioners, or even to testify before regional and state committees established to monitor MCO/HMO performance.

One role that the speech-language pathologist plays is that of the patient's communication advocate on transdisciplinary teams. This is especially crucial when one considers the treatment visit limits being imposed by insurers. Thus, the extent to which the clinician formulates a cogent, well-substantiated rationale regarding the need for speech-language pathology or audiological evaluation and treatment services significantly increases the likelihood that the patient will receive this treatment. In today's competitive environment, the communication disorders professional must be an assertive advocate on behalf of his or her clients/patients.

CONCLUSION

Access to and coverage of speech-language pathology services are the most critical challenges facing persons needing these services and their clinicians today. The increasing scarcity of health care resources means that speech-language pathologists must become more active advocates on behalf of their clients (Hallowell & Henri, 1997, 1998). Although the need for speech-language pathology services may seem obvious to the clinician, the speech-language pathology clinician must demonstrate to consumers, colleagues in other professions, referral sources, and MCOs/HMOs that these services are essential to the total care of a patient.

Discussion Questions

1. How does the increased focus on documenting clinical outcomes affect the types of patients who are eligible for services?
2. What actions might speech-language pathologists take to ensure that services are covered by payers?
3. How is the demand for clinical productivity changing the manner in which speech-language pathology services are delivered?
4. What skills must speech-language pathologists develop in order to be effective practitioners in the managed care environment?

REFERENCES

American Speech-Language-Hearing Association. (1994). “Code of Ethics.” *Asha, 36* (Suppl. 13), 1–2.

American Speech-Language-Hearing Association. (1996a). Guidelines for the training, credentialing, use, and supervision of speech-language pathology assistants. *Asha, 38* (Suppl. 16), 21–34.

American Speech-Language-Hearing Association. (1996b). Technical report of the Ad Hoc Committee on Multiskilling. *Asha, 38* (Suppl. 16), 53–61.

American Speech-Language-Hearing Association. (1997a). *Preferred practice patterns for the profession of audiology*. Rockville, MD: Author.

American Speech-Language-Hearing Association. (1997b). *Preferred practice patterns for the profession of speech-language pathology*. Rockville, MD: Author.

American Speech-Language-Hearing Association. (1997c). Position statement: Multiskilled personnel. *Asha, 39* (Suppl. 17), 13.

American Speech-Language-Hearing Association. (1997d). Technology 2000: Clinical applications for speech-language pathology. Rockville, MD: Author.

American Speech-Language-Hearing Association, Strategic Resources Group. (1991, November). Getting in shape: Lean cuisine for the ’90s. *Asha, 33* (11), 57–60.

American Speech-Language-Hearing Association, Task Force on Treatment Outcomes and Cost Effectiveness. (1995, November–December). Collecting outcome data: Existing tools, preliminary data, future directions, *Asha, 37* (11–12), 36–38.

American Speech-Language-Hearing Association, Task Force on Treatment Outcomes and Cost Effectiveness (1997, Winter). Treatment outcomes: Data for adults in health care environments. *Asha, 39* (1), 26–31.

Ashby, S.A. (1995, June–July). The renaissance professional: Doing more with less. *Asha, 37* (6–7), 33–36.

Breakey, L.K. (1994). Negotiating managed care contracts. In Ad Hoc Committee on Managed Care (Ed.), *Managing Managed Care* (pp. 21–28). Rockville, MD: American Speech-Language-Hearing Association.

Callahan, D. (1992). Symbols, rationality, and justice: Rationing health care. *American Journal of Law and Medicine, 18*, 1–13.

Clement, D.G., Retchin, S.M., Brown, R.S., & Stegall, M.H. (1994). Access and outcomes of elderly patients enrolled in managed care. *Journal of the American Medical Association, 271* (19), 1487–1492.

Cornett, B.S. (1994). Service delivery issues in health care settings. In R. Lubinski & C. Frattali (Eds.), *Professional issues in speech-language pathology and audiology* (pp. 188–200). San Diego, CA: Singular Publishing Group.

Des Rosier, M., Cantanzaro, M., & Piller, J. (1992). Living with chronic illness: Social support and the well spouse perspective. *Rehabilitation Nursing, 17*, 87–91.

Engelhard, C.L., & Childress, J.F. (1995, Winter–Spring). Caveat emptor: The cost of managed care. *Trends in Health Care, Law & Ethics, 10*, (1–2), 11–14, 71–72.

Evans, R., Bishop, D., & Haselkorn, J. (1991). Factors predicting satisfactory home care after stroke. *Archives of Physical and Medical Rehabilitation, 72*, 144–147.

Fisher, R.S. (1994, May). Medicaid managed care: The next generation? *Academic Medicine, 69* (5), 317–322.

Fox, H.B., Wicks, L.B., & Newacheck, P.W. (1993). State Medicaid health maintenance organization policies and special-needs children. *Health Care Financing Review, 15*, 25–37.

Frattali, C.M. (1990–1991). In pursuit of quality: Evaluating clinical outcomes. *National Student Speech Language Hearing Association Journal, 18*, 4–16.

Gerard, R. (1990). Preparing a multiskilled work force for the 21st century hospital. *Journal of Biocommunication, 17* (4), 24–26.

Gill, H.S. (1995, December). The changing nature of ambulatory rehabilitation programs and services in a managed care environment. *Archives of Physical Medicine and Rehabilitation, 76*, SC10–SC15.

Goldberg, B. (1996, Summer). Imagining tomorrow: What's ahead for our professions. *Asha, 38* (3), 23–28.

Goldberg, B. (1997, Fall). Linking up with telehealth. *Asha, 39* (4), 27–31.

Griffin, K.M., & Fazen, M. (1993, Winter). A managed care strategy for practitioners. *Quality Improvement Digest*, 1–7.

Hall, J.W. (1992). Intraoperative monitoring. *Handbook of auditory evoked responses* (pp. 509–533). Needham Heights, MA: Allyn and Bacon.

Hallowell, B., & Henri, B.P. (1997, September). *Constructive strategies for a new era in neurogenic communication disorders*. Seminar presented at the 25th Anniversary Conference of the Ohio Aphasiology Association, Columbus, OH.

Hallowell, B., & Henri, B.P. (1998, March). *Constructive advocacy under managed care.* Seminar presented at the annual convention of the Ohio Speech and Hearing Association, Akron, OH.

Hallowell, B., Henri, B.P., & Napp, A. (1997, April). *Actions for advocacy to address the challenges of managed care.* Workshop sponsored by the American Speech-Language-Hearing Association, Dallas, TX.

Hallowell, B., & Katz, R.C. (in press). Technological applications in the assessment of acquired neurogenic disorders in adults. *Seminars in Speech, Language, and Hearing, 20* (2).

Henri, B.P., & Cornett, B. (1992). Planning and documentation: Essential for quality and reimbursement. *Hearsay: Journal of the Ohio Speech and Hearing Association 7* (1), 12–15.

Henri, B.P., & Hallowell, B. (1996). Action planning for advocacy: Meeting managed care's challenges to speech-language pathology and audiology. *Hearsay: Journal of the Ohio Speech and Hearing Association, 11* (1), 40–42.

Henri, B.P., & Hallowell, B. (1997a, January). *Ethics, productivity and incentives: A synthesis for human service organizations.* Workshop presented to the Youngstown United Way Council of Agency Executives, Youngstown, OH.

Henri, B.P., & Hallowell, B. (1997b, October). Ethics and clinical productivity pressures under managed care. *Newsletter of Special Interest Division 11* 7 (3), 8 (Administration and Supervision, American Speech-Language-Hearing Association).

Hillman, A.L. (1995). The impact of physician financial incentives on high-risk populations in managed care. *Journal of Acquired Immune Deficiency Syndromes and Human Retrovirology, 8* (Suppl. 1), 523–530.

Hoen, B., Thelander, M.N., & Worsely, J. (1997). Improvement in psychosocial well-being of people with aphasia and their families: Evaluation of a community-based programme. *Aphasiology, 11,* 681–691.

Holzemer, W.L. (1996). The impact of multiskilling on quality of care. *International Nursing Review, 41* (1), 21–25.

Iglehart, J.K. (1995). Health policy report: Medicaid and managed care. *New England Journal of Medicine, 332* (25), 1727–1731.

Kahan, J.P., Bernstein, S.J., Leape, L.L., Hilborne, L.H., Park, R.E., Parker, L., Kamberg, C.J., & Brook, R.H. (1994). Measuring the necessity of medical procedures. *Medical Care, 32* (4), 357–365.

Keatley, M.A., Miller, T.I., & Mann, A. (1995, February). Treatment planning using outcome data: Fitting the pieces together. *Asha, 37* (2), 49–52.

Kidder, T.M., Langmore, S.E., & Martin, B.J.W. (1994). Indications and techniques of endoscopy in evaluation of cervical dysphagia: Comparison with radiographic techniques. *Dysphagia, 9,* 256–261.

Kimbarow, M.L. (1997, Fall). Ahead of the curve: Improving service with speech-language pathology assistants. *Asha, 39* (4), 41–44.

Leigh, W.A. (1994). Implications of health-care reform proposals for black Americans. *Journal of Health Care for the Poor and Underserved, 5* (1), 17–32.

Lyon, J.G. (1992, May). Communication use and participation for adults with aphasia in natural settings: The scope of the problem. *American Journal of Speech-Language Pathology, 1* (3), 7–14.

Mason, D.G. (1996). Quality of life for deaf and hard-of-hearing people. In Renwick, R., Brown, I., & Nagler, M. (Eds.), *Quality of life in health promotion and rehabilitation: Conceptual approaches, issues, and applications* (pp. 237–252). London: Sage Publications.

Mechanic, D. (1996). Changing medical organization and the erosion of trust. *Milbank Quarterly, 74* (2), 171–189.

Medicare HMOs with high rates of voluntary disenrollment fully accredited. (1998, Winter). *Health Advocate, 191,* 8.

Minifie, F.D. (1997). The educational continuum: A.A., B.A., M.A., Ph.D., Postdoctoral. *Proceedings of the eighteenth annual conference on graduate education* (pp. 8–19). Minneapolis: Council of Graduate Programs in Communication Sciences and Disorders.

Moore, M., & Rabins, A. (1996). Fed ax risks SLP, AUD jobs. *ASHA Leader, 1* (1), 1, 6.

National Center for Treatment Effectiveness in Communication Disorders. (1999, February). *Gaining the support of your staff and administration: Health Care* [On-line]. Available: www.asha.org/professionals/NCTECD/health.htm, 1–7.

Oberlander, J.B. (1997, April). Managed care and Medicare reform. *Journal of Health Politics, Policy and Law, 32* (2), 595–627.

O'Malley, J. (1997, March). Ethics and managed care. *Aspen's Advisor, 12* (3), 1–5.

Perkins, J. (1998, February). *Managed care update.* Los Angeles: National Health Law Program.

Perkins, J., & Olson, K. (1997, March). *Model medical necessity definition for physical care contracts.* Los Angeles: National Health Law Program.

Perkins, J., & Olson, K. (1998, Winter). The threat of evidence-based definitions of medical necessity. *Health Advocate, 91,* 17.

Pietranton, A.A., & Lynch, C. (1995, June–July). Multiskilling: A renaissance or a dark age? *Asha, 36* (6–7), 37–40.

Purtilo, R.B. (1995, Winter–Spring). Managed care: Ethical issues for the rehabilitation professions. *Trends in Health Care, Law & Ethics, 10,* 1–2, 105–108.

Records, N.L., Tomblin, J.B., & Freese, P.R. (1992). The quality of life of young adults with histories of specific language impairment. *American Journal of Speech-Language Pathology, 1,* 44–53.

Scott, A. (1998, January). Changes in compensation. *Advance, 8,* (2), 10–12.

Screen, M.R., & Anderson, N.B. (1994). Legal and ethical issues in communication disorders affecting multicultural populations. In *Multicultural perspectives in communication disorders* (pp. 51–64). San Diego, CA: Singular Publishing Group.

Smith, G., & Ashbaugh, J. (1995). *Managed care and people with developmental disabilities: A guidebook.* Alexandria, VA: National Association of State Directors of Developmental Disabilities, Inc., & the Human Services Research Institute.

Smith, E., Verdolini, K., Gray, S., Nichols, S., Lemke, J., Barkmeier, J., Dove, H., & Hoffman, H. (1996). Effect of voice disorders on quality of life. *Journal of Medical Speech-Language Pathology, 5,* 223–244.

Stenger, A. (1993, November). Who will advocate for patients? *Postgraduate Medicine, 94* (7), 108–110.

Swartz, K., & Brennan, T.A. (1996). Integrated health care, capitated payment, and quality: The role of regulation. *Annals of Internal Medicine, 124* (4), 442–447.

The threat of evidence-based definitions of medical necessity. (1998, Winter). *Health Advocate, 191,* 17.

Vekovius, G.Y. (1995, September). Managed care 101. *Asha, 37* (9), 45–47.

SUGGESTED READINGS

Ad Hoc Committee on Managed Care of the American Speech-Language-Hearing Association. (1994). *Managing managed care: A practical guide for speech-language pathologists & audiologists*. Rockville, MD: ASHA.

Knight, W. (1998). Managed care: What it is and how it works. Gaithersburg, MD: Aspen.

Kongstvedt, P. (1997). *Essentials of managed health care* (2nd. ed.). Gaithersburg, MD: Aspen.

Kreb, R., & Wolf, K. (1997). *Successful operations in the treatment-outcomes-driven world of managed care*. Rockville, MD: National Student Speech-Language-Hearing Association.

CHAPTER 2

Measuring and Managing Outcomes

Carol M. Frattali

Objectives

- Define relevant terms regarding outcomes.
- Cast outcomes in the conceptual framework of the World Health Organization's *International Classification of Impairments, Disabilities, and Handicaps.*
- Identify relationships across types of outcomes.
- Link the clinical process to client outcomes.
- Select appropriate outcome measures.
- Distinguish outcomes research from efficacy research.
- Apply a practical method to assess outcomes for individual clients.
- Manage outcomes to improve quality of care.

INTRODUCTION

From a managerial view, outcomes measurement and management have taken center stage in a service-delivery system driven by proof of value for dollars spent. The system, and its predominance of managed care, has focused its attention on matters of economic interest. Consider the following questions from a recent journal article addressing alternatives to conventional aphasia rehabilitation:

> Given that speech therapy may work for some patients. . . ; what is the cost-to-benefit ratio of the gains made? Do the gains made as a result of therapy translate into practical use that improves the

> patient's functional independence or quality of life? How does speech therapy compare in cost benefit with other potential uses of medical resources for these patients, e.g., personal care services, adaptive equipment, etc? (Weinrich, 1997, p. 107)

The clinical/research perspective offers a different angle. From this view, outcomes measurement and management have been steered by clinically and scientifically based concerns driven largely by the search for knowledge about which interventions work and which do not, and which work better than others. Olswang and Bain (1994, p. 55) capture this perspective: "Not having data concerning a client's progress during treatment is tantamount to being unprepared for a lecture, or showing up at a birthday party without a present—totally unthinkable."

Regardless of whether one's orientation is management, clinical practice, or research, outcomes measurement and management have become trademarks of contemporary care. The activities span a wide range of clinical and scientific methods—from nonexperimental to experimental research designs, and from a paper-and-pencil pretest/posttest for individual clients to aggregate data analysis using computerized management systems for large client populations.

This chapter defines relevant terminology and an evolving conceptual framework of client outcomes, addresses the decision-making process regarding which outcome measures to select, identifies available resources, offers a practical method for assessing outcomes with individual clients, and addresses the importance of outcomes management.

DEFINING RELEVANT TERMS

An outcome is a result of an intervention. There can be more than one outcome depending on whose perspective is taken into account (such as clinician, payer, administrator, client/family) and when measurement occurs (such as short-term, or long-term measurements). Donabedian (1980) defines the term *outcome* as:

> . . . a change in a patient's current and future health status that can be attributed to antecedent health care. Change includes improvement of social and psychological function in addition to the more usual emphasis on the physical and physiological aspects of

> performance. By still another extension, [change includes] patient attitudes (including satisfaction), health-related knowledge acquired by the patient, and health-related behavioral change. All of these can be seen either as components of current health or as contributions to future health. (pp. 82–83)

A clinical intervention, therefore, can result in different outcomes that reflect the range of perspectives of clients and other interested agents or consumers. When these perspectives are addressed together, categories and examples of outcomes can be generated as follows:

- *clinically derived*—ability to sustain phonation, accuracy in naming, type and frequency of disfluencies in a speech sample, integrity of the swallowing mechanism
- *functional*—ability to communicate basic needs, use the telephone, read the newspaper, eat independently
- *social*—employability, ability to learn, reintegration in community
- *patient-defined*—satisfaction with treatment; quality of life
- *administrative*—patient referral patterns, average length of stay, rate of missed sessions, productivity level in direct patient care
- *financial*—cost-effective care, cost benefit of care, rate of rehospitalizations, discharge destination

Casting Outcomes in a Conceptual Framework

Another way of thinking about outcomes is to cast them in an accepted framework of the consequences of a disease or disorder. The most common framework is the World Health Organization's (WHO's) *International Classification of Impairments, Disabilities, and Handicaps* (ICIDH) (WHO, 1980). This typology, which has been defined and used widely in the health care field for almost two decades, links the following chain of principal events that occur as the result of illness or injury:

1. Something abnormal happens (a pathology occurs).
2. Someone becomes aware of such an occurrence (recognition of an impairment).
3. The individual's performance or behavior may be altered and common activities may be restricted (giving rise to a disability).

4. The individual is placed at a disadvantage relative to others, thus socializing the experience (creating a handicap).

The chain of events can be applied to a communication or swallowing disorder, with an *impairment* defining specific speech, language, swallowing, or cognitive deficits; a *disability* encompassing the effects of the impairment(s) on everyday communicative or eating activities; and a *handicap* comprising a range of social effects as defined by a workplace or school system, family relationships, community roles, etc.

The ICIDH has been the subject of criticism in recent years (for its use of the outdated term *handicap*, its perceived oversight of the interrelationships across its classifications, and its biomedical focus), which prompted a revision of the model. Known as the ICIDH-2, the model is currently in development, and its classifications have been recast in order to approximate an acceptable common language for functioning and disablement (WHO, 1998). The revisions reflect a new social understanding of disability and describe the dimensions of functioning and disablement at three levels: the body, the person, and society. Definitions of these levels of functioning are:

- *impairment*—a loss or abnormality of body structure or of a physiological or psychological function (for example, loss of speech, loss of vision)
- *activity*—the nature and extent of functioning at the level of the person (such as taking care of oneself, communication activities, activities required of a job); activities may be limited in nature, duration, and quality
- *participation*—the nature and extent of a person's involvement in life situations in relation to impairment, activities, health conditions, and contextual factors (such as being employed, participating in community events, ability to vote). Participation may be restricted in nature, duration, and quality.

Table 2–1 presents an overview of the ICIDH-2.

The inclusion of contextual factors in the model addresses the social aspects of disablement and has strong implications for identification and removal of physical, environmental, and social barriers in order to enhance activities and participation. Thus, the ICIDH has evolved from a biomedical model focused on causation and cure, to an integrated biopsychosocial

Table 2–1 Overview of Dimensions of the ICIDH-2

	Impairments	*Activities*	*Participation*	*Contextual Factors*
Functioning	At body level	At person level	At social level	In interaction with environmental and personal factors
Characteristics	Body function, body structure	Person's daily activities	Involvement in the situation	Features of the physical, social, and attitudinal world
Positive aspect	Functional and structural integrity	Activity	Participation	Facilitators
Negative aspect	Impairment	Activity limitation	Participation restriction	Barriers

Source: Reprinted with permission from Toward A Common Language for Functioning and Disablement: ICIDH-2, The International Classification of Impairments, Activities, and Participation, Prefinal Draft, p. 11 © 1998, World Health Organization.

model of human functioning and disablement that extends its focus to removing barriers that interfere with activities of daily living and quality of life.

Examining Relationships across Classes of Outcomes

Although insufficient clinical research has been carried out to discern relationships across various outcomes, we do know that one-to-one relationships across outcomes are often the exception. In other words, we cannot assume that a severe impairment will result in severe activity limitations and, in turn, severe participation restrictions. The professional literature (as well as clinical experience) is replete with examples to the contrary. Enderby and John (1997), for example, describe two individuals, using the original ICIDH terminology, to illustrate the dynamic relationships inherent in outcomes. The first individual, Mr. K, has mild anomic aphasia. He cannot be understood easily in group conversations or over the telephone. He depends on others to be attentive and patient listeners. As a result of his aphasia and consequent difficulties in communicative interactions, Mr. K has lost his job, has withdrawn from social situations, and no longer contributes to family decision making. Mr. K, then, has a mild impairment, a moderate disability, and severe handicap. The second individual, Mrs. C, has cerebral palsy, is quadriplegic, and is severely dysarthric. She is totally independent, using an adapted wheelchair, and is living in an adapted environment. She can communicate in all situations using an Augmentative and Alternative Communication (AAC) system and special telephone adaptations. Despite her impairments, Mrs. C is employed as a health policy analyst, is an active member of society, and has a full work and social life. Her opinions are sought and valued in both work and social settings. Mrs. C has a severe impairment, no disability, and no handicap. These two examples underscore the importance of identifying and removing environmental and social barriers as a goal necessary for successful rehabilitation.

Holland (1998) describes a woman whom she evaluated four years after a stroke. This individual achieved an aphasia quotient of 18 on the Western Aphasia Battery (Kertesz, 1982), representing severe aphasia. Yet, this woman lives alone in a home she bought since her stroke, drives a car, and largely manages her own affairs. Her life skills were not predictable from her Western Aphasia Battery performance. Sarno (1965) believes that the ability to communicate, despite the presence of impairment, is bound by many contributory factors. She uses an example of the highly educated individual with a record of achievement whose communication needs differ from the individual with limited education and vocational goals. If these two individuals acquired similar speech impairments, they would likely exhibit differing degrees of disability and/or handicap, particularly on the job. Another example is two persons with severe verbal expressive impairment. One may experience only mild disability or no disability at all with adept use of an augmentative communication system; the other may be severely disabled, lacking access to an AAC system or being unable to use the system effectively.

In perhaps the first study to investigate the relationship between language and functional communication skills, Murray and colleagues (1984) tested the hypothesis that clients with Alzheimer's disease appear to have more communicative competence than they actually do, given their ability to talk fluently until the later stages of the disease; and that clients with aphasia appear to have less communicative competence than they actually do, given their impaired language abilities. They administered the Communicative Abilities in Daily Living (CADL) (Holland, 1980) to assess functional communication skills, and the Porch Index of Communicative Ability (PICA) (Porch, 1971) to assess language and communication skills of 10 subjects with aphasia and 10 subjects with dementia. They found that the dementia group scored significantly higher than did the aphasia group on the PICA, and the aphasia group scored significantly better than did the dementia group on CADL, thus confirming the hypothesized inverse relationship between functional communication and language skills.

Linking Process to Outcome

Despite the value and good sense inherent in measuring outcomes, a preoccupation with outcomes measurement to the exclusion of linking outcomes to antecedent contributory inputs and processes leads to serious research design flaws and misinterpretations of study results. An extreme example illustrating this danger is the outcomes study by the Health Care Financing Administration (HCFA) of the U.S. Department of Health and Human Services (Brinkley, 1986). In the mid 1980s, HCFA was pressured, as a result of the federal Freedom of Information Act, to publicly release death rates of hospitalized Medicare beneficiaries. Based on governmental predictions, 142 hospitals had significantly higher death rates, while 127 had significantly lower rates. One facility had a death rate of 86.7% compared to a predicted 22.5% death rate. Hospital administrators, angered by the data and subsequent media interpretations about quality of care, argued rightfully that HCFA failed to adjust adequately for risk of death. What the public did not know was that many hospitals with high mortality rates were tertiary-care centers treating more medically complex patients, and the facility with the most aberrant death rate was a hospice caring for terminally ill patients.

Donabedian's (1980) teachings are particularly relevant in light of the above example. His work was published during a time of intense debate over which approach—process or outcome assessment—was superior. He found, through conceptual and empirical study, that process and outcome are linked.

> Process and outcome are fundamentally linked in a single, symmetrical structure that makes of one almost a mirror image of the

> other, no matter how many attributes are used to test the relationship. Thus, the emphasis shifts to a more thorough understanding of the linkages between process and outcome, and away from the rather misguided argument over which of the two is the superior approach to assessment. (p. xi)

Donabedian's work may, indeed, have formed the foundation for development of outcomes management systems that adjust adequately for risk. The work of Iezzoni (1994) is particularly relevant to this topic, and interested readers are encouraged to refer to her book, *Risk Adjustment for Measuring Health Care Outcomes.*

WHICH MEASURES TO SELECT?

How does one choose among the growing number of outcome measures available? The logical first step would be to ask, "What is the purpose?" If the purpose is to investigate the benefit of treatment for an individual client, one should seek outcome measures that are both clinically sensitive and specific to the clinical condition. In line with ICIDH concepts that address impairments, activities, and participation, one might select a measure or set of measures designed to answer three questions:

1. Has the client's speech improved?
2. Is he or she a more functional communicator as a result?
3. Does the client feel better about himself/herself and less socially stigmatized?

The clinician chooses a measure or battery of measures to answer these three questions. A good resource for condition-specific outcome measures is a recent text devoted to the topic of outcomes measurement that contains chapters, written by experts in the field, on the following topics within the ICIDH or similar framework: culturally and linguistically diverse populations (Kayser, 1998); aphasia (Holland & Thompson, 1998); cognitive communication disorders resulting from traumatic brain injury (Adamovich, 1998), right-hemisphere brain damage (Tompkins & Lehman, 1998), and dementia (Bourgeois, 1998); dysphagia (Logemann, 1998); motor speech disorders (Beukelman, Mathy, & Yorkston, 1998); voice disorders (Verdolini,

Ramig, & Jacobson, 1998); fluency disorders (Blood & Conture, 1998); and child language and phonological disorders (Goldstein & Gierut, 1998).

Some individuals measure outcomes for managerial purposes to justify their worth as service providers and to safeguard their jobs. The questions change: Do speech-language pathology services benefit clients generally? Are the services cost-effective? In this context, one may decide to select a measure or set of measures that covers the case mix and that all speech-language pathologists in the organization can incorporate easily and quickly into their routine practice. A good choice would be a measure (preferably an automated system) that yields both cost and performance aggregate data in terms that managers can understand (for example, in terms of functional improvement). These types of measures may give less clinical information about individual clients but sufficient information for managerial purposes for client groups. These measures are appropriate for the following reasons:

- Measurement becomes uniform across clients and client groups, and clinicians can be trained to collect reliable data.
- Information can often be translated into a graded point rating system, which is used widely in the current service delivery system.
- Automated systems can pair financial data with performance data and compute the analyses (therefore, saving time).

A good review of automated outcomes management systems is provided by Keatley, Miller, and Johnson (1998). These authors cover the features of widely used systems, both for multidisciplinary rehabilitation and speech-language pathology, according to software developer, hardware requirements, applicable client populations, and system functions.

Finally, one's interest may be in collecting state and/or national outcomes data. One may, for instance, wish to know how a particular state or the nation looks with regard to treatment outcomes across the full range of clinical populations in all work settings. The purposes of this data collection effort may be:

- to convince legislators that a portion of health care and/or education dollars should be allocated to speech-language pathology services, therefore improving public access to these services
- to compare state performance to the national average as a benchmark of quality of care

This is an ambitious endeavor, involving perhaps a three- to five-year roll-out plan to institute outcomes measurement on a wide scale. The following steps are involved:

1. Create an organizational infrastructure to support, organize, and manage the effort.
2. Select an outcome measure or set of outcome measures that can easily be incorporated into clinical procedures and that span the full range of communication disorders and are applicable across the full range of work settings.
3. Identify a central data repository for data storage, organization, analysis, and reporting purposes.
4. Include in the database those variables that can influence outcomes (such as facility and clinician characteristics, client demographic characteristics). In this way, variations in performance can be explained.

The best resource for learning more about state- and national-level outcomes initiatives is the American Speech-Language-Hearing Association (ASHA) and its work, through the former ASHA Task Force on Treatment Outcomes and Cost Effectiveness and the current Center for Treatment Effectiveness, to collect national outcomes data. Readers are referred to Gallagher (1998) for a detailed chronology of this initiative, the outcomes measurement tools that are being used, and how to participate in this national project.

In summary, one's purposes will dictate selection of outcome measures. As the scope of the effort expands, sensitivity and specificity of measurement generally are compromised, which sometimes becomes an unavoidable trade-off.

A word or two needs to be said about the distinguishing features of outcomes research vis-à-vis efficacy research. The two are quite different both in design and in interpretation of research findings. Efficacy research involves highly controlled experimental conditions that allow the researcher to make statements about cause and effect. Thus, the outcomes of treatment are measured under *ideal* circumstances. Experimental methods include group designs and single-subject designs. In contrast, outcomes research involves quasi-experimental conditions (that is, it employs methods that adequately adjust for variables that can affect outcomes, such as age, severity of illness, and comorbidities) which allow the researcher to make statements about trends and associations. Therefore, the outcomes of treatment are measured under *typical* circumstances. While efficacy research often occurs under the controlled conditions of the laboratory, outcomes research occurs in the real world. Olswang (1998) provides an in-depth review of this topic.

THE TIMING OF MEASUREMENT

Outcomes can occur at various times either during or after the completion of a course of clinical intervention. Three terms have been used frequently in the field to classify the temporal aspects of outcomes: intermediate, instrumental, and ultimate outcomes (Rosen & Proctor, 1981). *Intermediate outcomes* determine, from session to session, whether treatment is benefiting the client. These outcomes allow investigation of the treatment process and can determine whether certain treatment methods (such as oral/facial exercises, head positioning) are necessary for adequate chewing and swallowing. *Instrumental outcomes* activate the learning process. These are outcomes that, when reached, trigger the ultimate outcome. Theoretically, once an instrumental outcome is reached, treatment is no longer necessary; the client will continue to improve on his or her own. *Ultimate outcomes* demonstrate the social or ecological validity of interventions, such as functional communication, reemployability, community reintegration, and individually defined quality of life (Frattali, 1998).

Outcomes data can be collected to investigate both the short-term and long-term effects of intervention. Although most would agree that long-term outcomes are a more important indicator of treatment benefit, they are the most difficult to measure objectively and accurately. First, clients can be lost to follow-up. Second, linking treatment to its long-term outcomes is more difficult when variables outside the control of the researcher (such as the effect of support networks, progression of disease, client motivation and coping skills, aging) fill the time gap. Third, longitudinal studies require considerable human and financial resources, which often are not supported by payers or administrators who are focused on quick results and immediate rather than future costs.

A PRACTICAL METHOD OF OUTCOMES ASSESSMENT FOR INDIVIDUAL CLIENTS

The clinical relevance of outcomes assessment is most apparent to clinicians who are faced daily with "proving their worth." But, clinical outcomes data supplied to decision makers are often subject to the "so what" question. So what if the client can repeat more words with greater accuracy? So what if the client can speak in complete sentences during a picture description task? So what if the client can match pictures to words? How do these skills make this person a more effective communicator who is better equipped to function in the real world?

In response to the various concerns surrounding outcomes assessment, staff from the Speech-Language Pathology Section of the National Institutes of Health (NIH) W.G. Magnuson Clinical Center developed a case review format from a publication on case studies in aphasia (Helm-Estabrooks & Holland, 1998). The NIH case review format (see Appendix 2–A) uses as its framework the ICIDH-2 model that classifies the consequences of disease—from body level, to person level, to society level. Outcome measures that are selected to address each of these areas are used at admission and discharge to document change in peformance.

The case that follows serves as an example. It was developed by Kimbrough-Glears (1998), a graduate student from the University of the District of Columbia, who was completing a clinical practicum at NIH. The patient in this case was seen for only a short period of therapy (five weekly sessions).

Background

The conceptual framework applied to this case was the ICIDH-2 typology that addresses a continuum of the consequences of a disease/disorder, including focus on a person's ability to function in his or her natural environments.

Patient

Biographical Information

The patient was a 49-year-old male of Ethiopian descent. Afar was his first language. He was divorced, had an adult daughter, and lived with his nephew. The patient held a PhD in history and had previously been employed as a university professor. He was retired due to illness.

Medical History

In 1984, the patient was diagnosed with early-onset idiopathic Parkinson's disease. He followed a progressive course with increasing tremor, rigidity, dystonia, and accompanying dysarthria. A computed tomography (CT) scan in 1994 revealed mild prominence of the ventricles and sulci. Magnetic resonance imaging (MRI) in 1995 was unremarkable. The patient's cognitive status was tested to be within normal limits. He had no history of smoking, drinking, or drug use. For the past year, the patient had been treated with a combination of amantadine and pergolide. Medications were continually adjusted to control right-upper-extremity and jaw dystonia.

Assessment

Procedures

At the impairment level, the following measures were taken: oral mechanism examination (Sonies et al., 1987), computerized speech analysis (Kay Elemetrics Corporation, 1994), and speech parameters ratings (Sonies & Scheib, 1994). The measures assessed the structure and function of the speech mechanism and provided both instrumental and perceptual analyses of speech characteristics.

At the activities level, the patient completed the Communication Effectiveness Survey (Beukelman, Mathy, & Yorkston, 1998) to assess functional communication in various natural contexts.

At the participation level, the patient completed the Short Form-36 of the Medical Outcome Study (Ware & Sherbourne, 1992) to provide an overall profile of physical and emotional health as related to quality of life.

Rationale for Test Selection

This combination of measures was selected to address the three classes of outcomes at the impairment, activities, and participation levels. The perspective of the patient was considered paramount at the activities and participation levels. Therefore, these measures were selected because they are self-administered. At the impairment level, there was interest in supporting perceptual ratings with instrumental ratings, thereby yielding sensitive, objective data. All measures provided quantitative data that could be interpreted by other professionals.

Findings

At the Impairment Level. On the oral mechanism examination, the patient presented with moderate right facial asymmetry with observable drooling at the right corner of his mouth. Mild to moderate weakness and range of motion of tongue and lips were noted, with weakness greater on the right side. Oral/facial dystonia was pronounced on the left.

Computerized speech analysis revealed moderately reduced speech diadochokinesis, mildly reduced breath support for speech with hoarse vocal quality, and slightly high habitual pitch level. Various parameters using computerized speech measures are listed in Table 2–2.

Speech parameters ratings were judged by the clinician as follows: moderately hoarse vocal quality with glottal fry, normal resonance, mild dysfluencies in connected speech, moderately low vocal intensity, fast rate of speech, monotone/monostress, moderately imprecise articulation, flat/masked facial expression.

At the Activities Level. The Communicative Effectiveness Survey yielded an overall score of 3.85 (of total 7), revealing moderate effects on functional communication in the areas of speaking to strangers, speaking on the telephone, speaking in the presence of noise, speaking with children, and speaking over an intercom system (such as at fast-food drive-throughs) .

At the Participation Level. The Short Form-36 (SF-36) revealed a physical functioning score of 70.00 (national average, 86.50), emotional health score of 100 (national average, 85.42), and emotional well-being score of 92.00 (national average, 76.38). These findings represent psychosocial adaptation to chronic illness despite physical restrictions.

Diagnosis

The patient presented with a moderate hypokinetic dysarthria primarily characterized by reduced vocal intensity, hoarse vocal quality, monotone/

Table 2–2 Initial Assessment Findings: Computerized Speech Measures

Parameter	*Performance*	*Normal Range (Based on Age/Gender)*	*Severity*	*Area Assessed*
Diadochokinetic rate: /pa/	2.60/second	5.0–7.1/second	Moderate	Rapid alternating speech movements
Maximum phonation	12.82 seconds	13.0–18.1 seconds	Mild	Breath support for speech
Percentage voicing	8.53%	100%	Severe	Parameter of voice quality
Fundamental frequency of voice	115.17 Hz	107–113 Hz	Slightly high	Habitual pitch

monostress, fast rate of speech with disfluencies, and imprecise articulation.

Effects on Functional Abilities/Quality of Life

The patient's motor speech impairment was having a moderate to severe impact on functional communication in the patient's natural environments, particularly when speaking with strangers or on the telephone. Despite the level of speech impairment and activities limitations in functional communication, the patient presented an optimistic and upbeat approach to life as represented by high scores in emotional health and well-being.

Prognosis

The patient was considered a candidate for treatment on the basis of the following positive prognostic indicators: motivation, positive life outlook, stimulability to compensatory techniques, educational level, support system of family and friends. The prognosis for improvement at the impairment level was considered poor on the basis of the early onset of Parkinson's disease and the progressive nature of the disease.

Expected Outcomes

The clinician developed the following list of expected outcomes:

- *Impairment level.* The patient will increase his speech intelligibility as measured by improvements in breath support for speech and percentage of voicing during maximum phonation tasks on computerized speech measures and perceptual ratings of vocal intensity during speech tasks.
- *Activities level.* The patient will improve his communication effectiveness over the telephone, with strangers, and in noisy environments as measured by the Communication Effectiveness Survey.
- *Participation level.* The patient will participate in a wider range of social activities as measured by patient report. (*Note:* Because SF-36 findings represented good emotional health and well-being, there was no need to strive for these improvements as an outcome of therapy.)

Focusing Treatment

Methods

The treatment method involved utilization of pausing at natural phrase points and projecting voice to increase speech intelligibility. Treatment tasks followed a hierarchical progression from reading; to monologue; to spontaneous conversation in a quiet, one-on one setting; to a noisy, one-on-one setting; to a noisy group setting (cafeteria); and finally, to telephone conversation.

Rationale

The method is based on an approach to dysarthria that begins with the lowest subsystem (respiratory) and moves upwards (in this case, phonatory) to increase intelligibility (Dworkin, 1991).

Outcome Measures

Pre- and posttreatment outcome measures were the same measures used as initial assessment procedures. Session-to-session outcome measures included clinician ratings of intelligibility (as calculated by percentage of speech segments between pauses that were understood by the listener) in various speaking tasks.

Results of Treatment

Among the positive outcomes noted when using the compensatory techniques of pausing and projecting voice were the following findings:

- At the impairment level, the patient increased percentage of voicing on a computerized maximum phonation task from 8.53% at pretreatment to 30.15% at posttreatment (with sustained phonation at approximately 12 seconds at both pre- and posttreatment), indicating a stronger voice with decreased hoarseness. This difference was noted also in perceptual ratings of speech parameters, with vocal quality improving from 3 at pretreatment to 2.5 at posttreatment, and vocal intensity improved from 3 to 2.5. Perceptual ratings of intelligibility also improved from 3 to 2.
- At the activities level, the major area of improvement was noted in the domain of speaking over the telephone, as documented on the Communicative Effectiveness Survey. On a 7-point scale, with 7 being very effective, the patient rated his effectiveness in this communicative context from 2 at pretreatment to 4 at posttreatment. This patient-rated behavior was substantiated by session-to-session ratings by the clinician, averaging 80% speech intelligibility in telephone tasks.
- At the participation level, a readministration of the SF-36 revealed somewhat lower ratings than at pretreatment, documenting the fluctuations in physical abilities due to on-and-off conditions related to medications. The same relationship of physical to emotional health, however, was maintained (from 70 to 45 in physical health; from 100 to 95 in emotional health). In terms of social activities, the patient reported that he started using the telephone more and that he continued to receive feedback from listeners suggesting that he was easier to understand.

Discussion

This case suggests that a short, direct treatment regimen focused on compensatory techniques in the face of a degenerative disease at the chronic stage can be provided as an alternative to "ideal care" in the wake of changes imposed by managed health care. The case also suggests that a continuum of patient outcomes at the impairment, activities, and participation levels can be achieved and be perceived as beneficial to patients in common communication activities in natural contexts (such as telephone use).

"MANAGING" OUTCOMES

At the client level and the clinical population level, outcomes data must be managed if one is to improve the quality of care. The concept of using outcomes for decision making forms the core of Ellwood's (1988) approach to outcomes management. Providers may find that the costs of certain clinical procedures do not justify the minimal progress made with certain client populations, especially when less costly alternatives to treatment (such as family instruction or group or computer treatments) may have comparable results (Frattali, 1998). In this case, a decision can be made to allocate more resources to underserved client populations in which significant improvements can be documented.

Ellwood (1988) describes outcomes management as follows:

> . . . a technology of patient experience designed to help patients, payers, and providers make rational [health care–related] choices based on better insight into the impact of these choices on the patient's life. Outcomes management consists of the following:
>
> - a common patient-understood language of health outcomes
> - a national database containing clinical, financial, and health outcome information and analysis that estimates as best we can the relationship between [health care] interventions and health outcomes, as well as the relationship between health outcomes and money
> - an opportunity for each decision maker to have access to those analyses that are relevant to the choices they must make (p. 4)

At the clinical population level, management of outcomes allows the development of data-based standards of care and clinical management tools such as critical paths (treatment regimes supported by efficacy and outcomes research, which include only those vital elements that have been proved to positively influence patient outcomes) to improve the effectiveness and efficiency of care. At the individual client level, management of outcomes leads to necessary adjustments to the plan of care, and possibly treatment alternatives, to optimize the result of care as it is being provided.

CONCLUSIONS

This chapter defines relevant terminology and a new conceptual framework that provides a useful structure for measuring outcomes. It addresses the basic considerations inherent in selecting outcome measures, identifies available resources, offers a practical clinical method of measuring outcomes for use with individual clients, and addresses the importance of outcomes management. However, once the clinician masters skills of outcomes measurement and management, one will undoubtedly be left short-changed. That is because even the most sensitive and psychometrically sound outcome measures fails to detect insights yielded from keen clinical observations or a sharpened sixth sense of behavioral change.

Muriel Lezak (1989) offers good advice on the use of clinical tests, which can be adapted to the use of outcomes measures:

> [Outcomes measures] are simply a means of enhancing our observations. They can be thought of as extensions of our organs of perception—the seven-league boots of clinical behavioral observation. If we use them properly, . . . like seven-league boots they enable us to accomplish much more with greater speed. When tests are misused as substitutes for rather than extensions of clinical observations, they can obscure our view of the patient, much like seven-league boots would get in the way if worn over the head.

Consistent with this line of thinking, Wendell Johnson (1946) once said, "The map is not the territory." This maxim can be applied to outcomes measurement. In the realm of human communication, with all its nuances, complexities, and mysteries, even the best measures will fall short of expectations.

Discussion Questions

1. What are the various types of outcomes and how are they linked?
2. How are the new World Health Organization classifications of impairment, activity, and participation related?
3. What factors must be considered in selecting appropriate outcome measures?
4. How are outcomes "managed"?

REFERENCES

Adamovich, B.L.B. (1998). Outcome measurement in cognitive communication disorders, Section 1. Traumatic brain injury. In C.M. Frattali (Ed.), *Measuring outcomes in speech-language pathology* (pp. 334–353). New York: Thieme Medical Publishers.

Beukelman, D.R. (1998). Communication Effectiveness Survey. In Beukelman, D.R., Mathy, P., & Yorkston, K. (1998). Outcomes measurement in motor speech disorders. In C.M. Frattali (Ed.), *Measuring outcomes in speech-language pathology* (pp. 334–353). New York: Thieme Medical Publishers.

Beukelman, D.R., Mathy, P., & Yorkston, K. (1998). Outcomes measurement in motor speech disorders. In C.M. Frattali (Ed.), *Measuring outcomes in speech-language pathology* (pp. 334–353). New York: Thieme Medical Publishers.

Blood, G.W., & Conture, E.G. (1998). Outcomes measurement issues in fluency disorders. In C.M. Frattali (Ed.), *Measuring outcomes in speech-language pathology* (pp. 387–405). New York: Thieme Medical Publishers.

Bourgeois, M. (1998). Outcomes measurement in cognitive communication disorders: Section 3. Dementia. In C.M. Frattali (Ed.), *Measuring outcomes in speech-language pathology* (pp. 292–320). New York: Thieme Medical Publishers.

Brinkley, J. (1986, March 12). U.S. releasing lists of hospitals with abnormal mortality rates. *New York Times*, p. 1.

Donabedian, A. (1980). *Explorations in quality assessment and monitoring. Volume 1: The definition of quality and approaches to its assessment.* Ann Arbor, MI: Health Administration Press.

Dworkin, J.P. (1991). *Motor speech disorders: A treatment guide.* St Louis, MO: Mosby-Year Book.

Ellwood, P. (1988). Shattuck Lecture—Outcome management: A technology of patient experience. *New England Journal of Medicine, 318* (23), 1549–1556.

Enderby, P., & John, A. (1997). Therapy outcome measures: speech and language therapy. London: Singular Publications.

Frattali, C.M. (1998). Outcomes assessment in speech-language pathology. In A.F. Johnson & B.H. Jacobson (Eds.), *Medical speech-language pathology: A practitioner's guide* (pp. 685–709). New York: Thieme Medical Publishers.

Gallagher, T.M. (1998). National initiatives in outcomes measurement. In C.M. Frattali (Ed.), *Measuring outcomes in speech-language pathology* (pp. 527–557). New York: Thieme Medical Publishers.

Goldstein, H., & Gierut, J. (1998). Outcomes measurement in child language and phonological disorders. In C.M. Frattali (Ed.), *Measuring outcomes in speech-language pathology* (pp. 406–437). New York: Thieme Medical Publishers.

Helm-Estabrooks, N., & Holland, A. (1998). *Approaches to the treatment of aphasia.* San Diego, CA: Singular Publishing Group.

Holland, A.L. (1980). *Communicative abilities in daily living.* Baltimore: University Park Press.

Holland, A.L. (1998). Functional outcome assessment of aphasia following left hemisphere stroke. *Seminars in speech and language.* New York: Thieme Medical Publishers, 19 (3), pp. 249–260.

Holland, A.L., & Thompson, C.K. (1998). Outcomes measurement in aphasia. In C.M. Frattali (Ed.), *Measuring outcomes in speech-language pathology* (pp. 245–266). New York: Thieme Medical Publishers.

Iezzoni, L.I. (1994*). Risk adjustment for measuring health care outcomes.* Ann Arbor, MI: Health Administration Press.

Johnson, W. (1946). *People in quandaries: The semantics of personal adjustment.* New York: Harper & Row Publishers.

Kay Elemetrics Corporation. (1994). Computerized Speech Lab, Model 4300B, Software version, 5.X. Lincoln Park, NJ.

Kayser, H. (1998). Outcome measurement in culturally and linguistically diverse populations. In C.M. Frattali (Ed.), *Measuring outcomes in speech-language pathology* (pp. 225–244). New York: Thieme Medical Publishers.

Keatley, M.A., Miller, T.I., & Johnson, A.F. (1998). Designing automated outcomes management systems. In C.M. Frattali (Ed.), *Measuring outcomes in speech-language pathology* (pp. 186–208). New York: Thieme Medical Publishers.

Kertesz, A. (1982). *Western Aphasia Battery: Test manual.* San Antonio, TX: The Psychological Corporation.

Kimbrough-Glears, D. (1998). Case presentation: Treating dysarthria in Parkinson's disease. Presented at Rehabilitation Grand Rounds, National Institutes of Health, W.G. Magnuson Clinical Center, Bethesda, MD.

Lezak, M. (1989). In I.E. Asher (Ed.), Occupational assessment tools: An annotated index, 2nd ed. New York: Soho Press.

Logemann, J.A. (1998). Efficacy, outcomes, and cost effectiveness in dysphagia. In C.M. Frattali (Ed.), *Measuring outcomes in speech-language pathology* (pp. 321–333). New York: Thieme Medical Publishers.

Murray, J., Marquardt, T.P., Richardson, A., & Nalty, D. (1984). Differential diagnosis of aphasia and dementia from aphasia test battery scores. *Journal of Neurological Communication Disorders, 1*, 33–39.

Olswang, L.B. (1998). Treatment efficacy research. In C.M. Frattali (Ed.), *Measuring outcomes in speech-language pathology* (pp. 134–150). New York: Thieme Medical Publishers.

Olswang, L.B., & Bain, B. (1994). Data collection: Monitoring children's treatment progress. *American Journal of Speech-Language Pathology, 3* (3), 55–66.

Porch, B. (1971). *Porch index of communicative ability.* Palo Alto, CA: Consulting Psychologists Press.

Rosen, A., & Proctor, E. (1981). Distinctions between treatment outcome and their implications for treatment evaluation. *Journal of Consulting and Clinical Psychology, 49,* 418–425.

Sarno, M.T. (1965). A measurement of functional communication in aphasia. *Archives of Physical Medicine and Rehabilitation, 46*, 101–107.

Sonies, B.C., & Scheib, D. (1994). Speech parameters ratings. Bethesda, MD: National Institutes of Health, W.G. Magnuson Clinical Center.

Sonies, B.C., Weiffenbach, J., Atkinson, J.C., Brahim, J., Macynski, A., & Fox, P.C. (1987). Clinical examination of motor and sensory functions of the adult oral cavity. *Dysphagia, 1,* 178–186.

Tompkins, C.A., & Lehman, M.T. (1998). Outcome measurement in cognitive communication disorders, Section 2. Right hemisphere brain damage. In C.M. Frattali (Ed.), *Measuring outcomes in speech-language pathology* (pp. 281–291). New York: Thieme Medical Publishers.

Verdolini, K., Ramig, L., & Jacobson, B. (1998). Outcomes measurement in motor speech disorders. In C.M. Frattali (Ed.), *Measuring outcomes in speech-language pathology* (pp. 354–386). New York: Thieme Medical Publishers.

Ware, J., & Sherbourne, C. (1992). The MOS 36–item short form health survey (SF-36). *Medical Care, 30*, 473–483.

Weinrich, M. (1997). Computer rehabilitation in aphasia. *Clinical Neuroscience, 4*, 103–107.

World Health Organization. (1980). *International classification of impairments, disabilities, and handicaps*. Geneva: Author.

World Health Organization. (1998). *Toward a common language for functioning and disablement: ICIDH-2, The international classification of impairments, activities, and participation*. Prefinal draft. Geneva: Author.

SUGGESTED READINGS

American Speech-Language-Hearing Association. (1996). *A practical guide to applying treatment outcomes and efficacy resources*. Rockville, MD: Author.

Frattali, C. (Ed.). (1998). *Measuring outcomes in speech-language pathology*. New York: Thieme Medical Publishers.

Frattali, C. (Ed.). (1998). Assessing functional outcomes in neurogenic populations. *Seminars in Speech and Language, 19* (3).

Appendix 2–A National Institutes of Health Format for Case Reviews

I. Background
   A. Application of conceptual/theoretical model and pertinent clinical research to this case
   B. Definitions of relevant terminology
II. Patient
   A. Biographical information
   B. Medical history/pertinent medical test findings
III. Assessment
   A. Assessment procedures
   B. Rationale for selection of tests/measures
   C. Findings
IV. Diagnosis
   A. Impairment level/severity (e.g., aphasia, dysphagia, dysarthria/ mild, moderate, severe)
      1. Association with medical findings/pathophysiology
V. Effects on functional abilities/quality of life
   A. Effects of impairment on
      1. Activities/activities limitation (e.g., functional communication/eating meals)
      2. Participation/participation restriction (e.g., role changes, psychosocial effects, effect on school, work, family, community)
VI. Prognosis
   A. Prognostic indicators
      1. Positive
      2. Negative
VII. Expected outcomes
   A. Expected treatment outcomes (treatment goals)
      1. Impairment level (e.g., increased word retrieval, increased strength of oral/facial musculature, improvement in speech intelligibility)
      2. Activities level (e.g., functional communication)

3. Participation level (e.g., resolution of social isolation, depression; return to work/school; community reentry)

VIII. Focusing Treatment
   A. Methods
   B. Rationale for selection of methods (based on theoretical model, treatment efficacy literature)
   C. Outcome measures of impairment, activities, participation
      1. Pre-, interim-, post-treatment measures
      2. Other measures (e.g., interim, session-to-session)

IX. Results of treatment
   A. *Impairment level:* Modality-specific behaviors
   B. *Activities level:* Functional status (related to everyday life activities)
   C. *Participation level:* Quality of life (related to psychosocial status/adjustment, role changes, school/work/community involvement)

X. Discussion
   A. Lessons learned
   B. Treatment alternatives
   C. Realism (e.g., cost effectiveness, patient and family perceptions and satisfaction, applicability to other patients)

REFERENCE

Helm-Estabrooks, N., & Holland, A.L. (1998). Approaches to the treatment of aphasia. In R.T. Wertz (Series Ed.) Clinical competence series. San Diego, CA: Singular Publishing.

CHAPTER 3

Structuring Clinical Practice: Guidelines, Pathways, and Protocols

Becky Sutherland Cornett and Tracy L. Davidson

Objectives

- Understand the science of clinical practice and be able to apply principles to everyday services.
- Link evidence-based practice to principles of managed care.
- Differentiate among types of structured care methodologies.
- Develop appropriate structured care methodologies for use in clinical practice.
- Link outcomes measurement and management concepts to the use of structured care methodologies.
- Apply principles of disease management to the practice of speech-language pathology.

INTRODUCTION

In an era of rapid reforms in health care and education, speech-language pathologists and other practitioners in all work settings are being asked to demonstrate the value of their services by payers, regulators, and the public. Clinicians are facing numerous challenges, including the following:

- meeting policy makers' demands for efficient and effective allocation of resources to improve the overall health of the population
- facing payers' demands for clinical accountability

- responding to consumer demands for informed choice and treatment selection based on their needs, preferences, and desired outcomes
- determining methods of evaluating and selecting cost-effective service-delivery alternatives that demonstrate collaboration with other professionals
- responding to employers' pressure to meet the "bottom line"
- establishing best-practice standards for services based on scientific evidence
- using technology to collect, store, retrieve, analyze, and use clinical information

The purpose of this chapter is to help clinicians to meet the challenges presented here by offering tools and techniques that facilitate clinical practice management. Clinical guidelines and their companion documents—clinical pathways, protocols, and other resources—are intended to provide guidance in clinical decision making, to help determine best-practice standards, and to demonstrate the efficiency and effectiveness of patient care. The chapter discusses how these clinical tools are part of the science of practice (the principles) followed by definitions, examples, and everyday use of these documents (the practicalities). Next, the chapter provides information about the American Speech-Language-Hearing Association's (ASHA's) continuum of practice documents. The chapter concludes with a discussion of new applications of structuring care, including disease management and demand management.

PRINCIPLES OF STRUCTURED CARE: THE SCIENCE OF CLINICAL PRACTICE

Although clinical practice has always been tied to scientific inquiry, the environment of the current health care system has brought increased attention to the selection of treatment procedures based on the evidence of their value to achieve results. O'Neil (1998) summarizes the relationship between the managed care marketplace and science particularly well:

> Does anyone really desire unmanaged care? That is, care that would be delivered without attention to established guidelines based on empirical evidence, care that is wasteful of resources, or services that fail to meet basic consumer needs. Are we really

> concerned that a systematic approach to delivering services might affect quality care—care that is based on improving outcomes and holding providers accountable for those outcomes? And if accountability and outcomes are held constant or improved, does it matter that those services cost less under managed care? (p. 2)

Evidence-based practice is today's term for linking evaluation and treatment methods to science. *Webster's Unabridged Dictionary* defines science as "systematized knowledge derived from observation, study, and experimentation" and is completely consistent with O'Neil's call for a systematic approach to service delivery—to managing care based upon evidence. The system follows from the science. Domholdt (1997) contends that being guided by evidence requires the following: (1) literature that provides answers to common practice questions, (2) practitioners who study the literature and use it for clinical decision making, (3) colleagues who debate the literature together, and (4) clinicians who change their practices in light of new information.

The federal Agency for Health Care Policy and Research (AHCPR), which in the past used expert panels to develop nationally recognized clinical practice guidelines, has redirected its efforts to establish evidence-based practice centers, a national guidelines database, and research and evaluation services. AHCPR serves as a resource for organizations to develop their own guidelines. The purpose of the evidence-based practice centers is to provide extensive literature review on assigned topics and to produce "evidence reports" or technology assessments so that clinicians can make critical health care decisions based upon the latest and most comprehensive scientific knowledge. The evidence reports will become building blocks for health care quality improvement projects across the country (AHCPR, 1997). More information about AHCPR's efforts can be found at the following Web site: http://www.ahcpr.gov/.

As part of AHCPR's clinical practice guideline development process, levels of evidence for judging recommendations for inclusion of particular procedures or services (such as whether stroke patients should receive a swallowing evaluation) were used to determine their value to patient care (Stason, 1997). These levels of evidence are included here for reference.

- *Level A*: Recommendation is supported by two or more randomized controlled trials (RCTs) that specifically address the question of interest in a group of patients comparable to the one to which the recommendation applies.

- *Level B:* Recommendation supported by a single RCT meeting level-A criteria, by two or more RCTs that indirectly address the question of interest, or by two or more case control or cohort studies with multivariate analyses that control for group differences.
- *Level C*: Recommendation supported by a single, nonrandomized controlled trial meeting level B criteria or by two or more studies using historical controls or quasi-experimental designs.

According to Kreb and Wolf (1997), practice guidelines emerge from evidence-based practice, and their use requires that clinicians develop collaborative behaviors and new attitudes toward the role of science in practice—what Cornett and Chabon (1988) call a "scientific attitude." Kamhi (1984) argues that clinicians should be "clinical scientists," approaching clinical problem solving with the same skills as a researcher approaches a problem, including the formulation, testing, confirmation or refutation, and reformulation of hypotheses. Levenson's (1996) delineation of "essential care processes" is a particularly helpful example of a scientific approach to treatment. Using Levenson's model, the clinician systematically collects and analyzes data, incorporating practice guidelines, pathways, and other clinical tools to plan and manage care. Levenson's processes and objectives are found in Table 3–1. This approach reflects a commitment to clinical accountability in which the clinician follows a process of continuous review and justification of professional activities in terms of clinical and financial outcomes of care (Douglass, 1983). It is a matter of answering Douglass's (1983) timeless question: "How do we know, and how can we show that what we do in therapy makes a difference?" (p. 117).

Making a difference in the everyday lives of patients or clients is the ultimate goal of outcomes management efforts across the country. Outcomes management refers to the evaluation, analysis, and dissemination of the results of health care services in an effort to improve those outcomes. Outcomes management activities seek to identify optimal process-outcome linkages so that clinicians can manage for results. Paul Ellwood was among the first practitioners to emphasize the need for clinicians to quantify and qualify what they do to determine if their services achieve the desired health care outcomes. Ellwood (1988) defined outcomes management as a "technology of patient experience designed to help patients, payers, and providers make rational medical care-related choices based on

Table 3–1 Essential Care Processes

Process	*Objectives*
Assessment	• Collect information about the individual that allows proper definition of his/her problems.
Problem definition	• Correctly and completely define the individual's problems and needs, so that the appropriate care plan can be developed.
Cause-and-effect analysis	• Appropriately link various problems and diagnoses to their causes, as a basis for determining relevant treatments and services.
Identifying care goals and objectives	• Correctly and completely define the purpose of giving care and the criteria that will be used to determine when the objectives have been met.
Care planning	• Create a plan to address the individual's problems, including the responsibilities of various individuals and disciplines.
Management of identified problems and risks	• Identify and implement appropriate treatment alternatives to address the individual's primary (main reason for admission) and secondary (coexisting) problems and risks.
Management of new problems/complications	• Identify and manage problems that arise from existing conditions or that did not exist previously.
Prevention of nosocomial/iatrogenic problems	• Identify the areas of high risk and potential problems that arise as a result of medications and treatments, or by being in a health care facility, and institute measures to prevent those problems and to recognize them if they arise.
Preparation for completion of treatment course (where relevant)	• Monitor responses to treatment and progress toward discharge or completion of an episode of illness. • Plan for discharge and transfer by ensuring appropriate transfer site, follow-up of problems, and communication of information to the individual and family, and others who will be providing continuing care.
Follow-up	• Review outcomes for the episode or stay • Review problems and concerns based on input of the providers and recipients of the care.

Courtesy of American Medical Directors Association, Columbia, Maryland. The American Medical Directors Association is a national professional organization representing physicians who care for patients in long-term care settings as attending physicians and as medical directors. To obtain a list of AMDA publications, call the national office of AMDA at (800) 876-2632.

better insight into the effect of these choices on the patient's life" (p. 1551). He suggested the following four techniques to accomplish this broad task:

1. the development of clinical standards and guidelines to facilitate selection of appropriate interventions
2. the systematic measurement of patient functioning and well-being at appropriate time intervals
3. development of national databases of clinical and outcomes data
4. analysis and dissemination of results from the database

Similarly, Spath (1994) suggests that outcomes management can be achieved by concentrating on the following elements:

- *Outcomes specification:* Define expected outcomes and measures to assess achievement of results.
- *Outcomes measurement:* Design valid and reliable assessment tools.
- *Information systems:* Design automated or manual information systems to support data collection, input, retrieval, and analysis.
- *Process improvement:* Design continuous quality improvement techniques to improve the processes of care.

Wojner (1997a) describes the provider's perspective on outcomes management as an "ongoing quest for best practice" (p. 78). From the payer's perspective, outcomes management facilitates the prediction of resource use by offering a planned course of care based on clinical research to identify appropriate practices and continuous quality monitoring to improve efficiency.

Clinical guidelines and their companion documents or structured care methodologies (Merry, 1995; Wojner, 1997a) are outcomes management tools because they enhance practitioners' ability to quantify what they do and to select strategies to achieve specific results. Structured care methodologies, also called clinical decision support tools (Jacobs, 1997) and care management tools (Harvey & DePue, 1997a), provide a systematic methodology for defining, measuring, and improving clinical quality (Spath, 1994). These tools help to answer tough questions from multiple audiences seeking to divide today's scarce health care dollars. Structured or planned care does not preclude creativity in clinical practice; practitioners do not have to sacrifice "art" to achieve "science." However, they would do well to heed Wojner's (1997a) advice: "As health care providers today are faced with the challenge of providing care in an efficient and cost-effective manner, it is of paramount importance to let science guide bedside decisions" (p. 82).

THE PRACTICALITIES OF STRUCTURED CARE

The chapter turns now from discussing the principles of structured care to presenting the methods of accomplishing that care. Structured care methodologies are tools that help clinicians to define a course of treatment as part of a case management strategy. Case management might be thought of as individualized outcomes management. That is, case management efforts for specific patients help clinicians to achieve overall organizational outcomes management goals.

Case management is a collaborative process that assesses, plans, implements, coordinates, monitors, and evaluates the options and services required to meet an individual's health needs, using communication among professionals, payers, and patients and available resources to promote high-quality, cost-effective outcomes (Ray, 1998). According to the Joint Commission on Accreditation of Healthcare Organizations (Joint Commission) (1998), the goals of case management also include intervention at key points or significant variances for individual patients, and resolution of patterns of aggregate variances that have a negative quality-cost impact. Structured care methodologies (particularly clinical pathways) are used by case managers and patient care team members to facilitate the achievement of predictable outcomes. They allow for individualized plans of care while maintaining a systematic approach to treatment across a given diagnosis. Spath (1994) calls clinical pathways a "short-hand version" of the larger case management plan, which includes clinical problems and diagnoses, intermediate outcomes, discharge outcomes, clinical interventions, and estimated length of stay. The pathway functions as a reminder list of the care plan, specifying who is accountable for the care, time frames for completion of procedures and treatments, and expected outcomes of care (Mahn & Heller, 1994).

The concept of using pathways in health care was adapted from the critical path method used by engineers in the oil refinery, construction, and computer industries as a time management technique. The idea is to track and time precisely the critical points in completing projects (McDermott & Toerge, 1994). Intensive care unit nurses led by Karen Zander at the New England Medical Center first used clinical pathways in 1985 as a case management tool. As management tools, pathways organize, sequence, and time team interventions for a particular type of patient. They help caregivers "do the right thing the first time" for the patient (Spath, 1995, p. 26).

Structured care methodologies can be an important part of a health care organization's performance management process. Both Spath (1995) and Shekim (1994) used the Shewhart-Deming Plan-Do-Check-Act (PDCA) cycle to illustrate the role of guidelines and pathways in continuous quality improvement activities. This cycle is presented in Figure 3–1. According

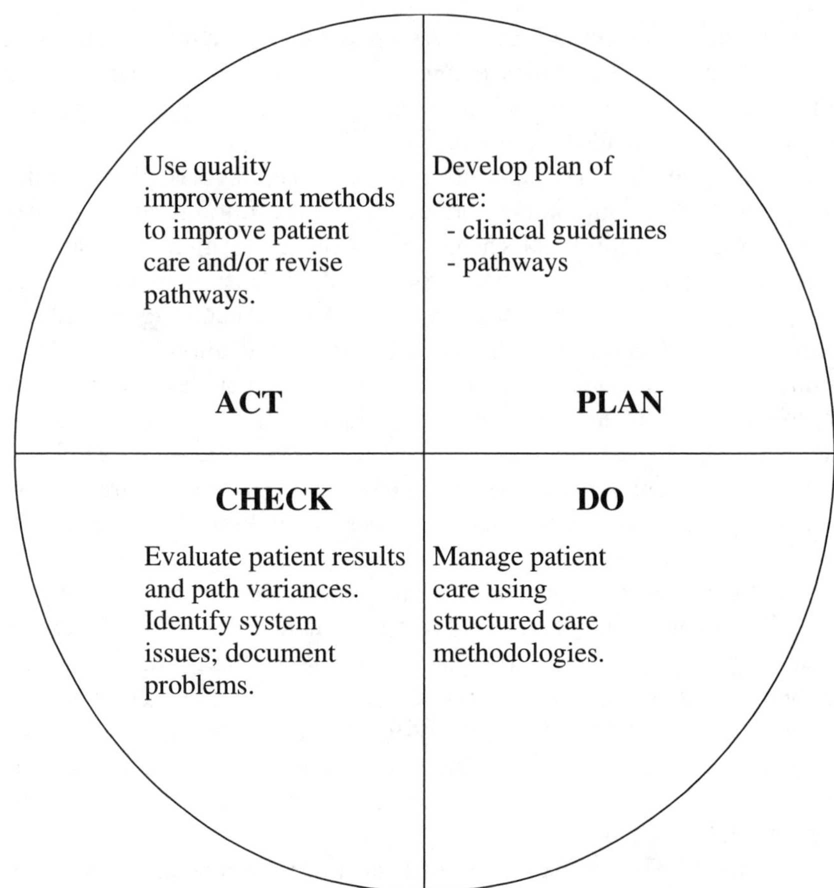

Figure 3–1 The Shewhart-Deming continuous process improvement cycle related to structured care methodologies.

Courtesy of American Speech-Language-Hearing Association, Rockville, Maryland.

to Shekim, pathways represent the plan of care, which reflects the team's ideal course of treatment for the patient. The actual interventions are the "do" part of the process improvement cycle. Clinicians consult clinical decision tools to determine what should be occurring (Spath, 1995). The "check" portion of the cycle includes evaluation of outcomes, analysis of the types of variances that may occur, and documentation of issues addressed. A variance is any difference between what was planned and what actually happened. Sources of variance may be related to the patient's condition, psychosocial issues, family problems, caregiver behaviors, or health care system errors. Variance analysis should guide the "act" part of the process improvement cycle, in which patient care services are continually evaluated and care plans are revised as the evidence indicates. More information about quality improvement processes can be found in Frattali (1998); Frattali and Cornett (1994); and McLaughlin and Kaluzny (1994). ASHA has also published books and materials about quality improvement, which are available by contacting the organization's product sales department.

Terms associated with structured care methodologies are often used interchangeably (for example, critical pathway, clinical pathway, care path, clinical guideline, protocol). Each methodology has a distinct definition, although they are closely related and complementary (Wojner, 1997b). Exhibit 3–1 features definitions of and relationships among clinical practice guidelines, algorithms, clinical pathways, and other companion documents. Field and Lohr (1992) and AHCPR (1995a, 1995b) provide detailed information about clinical guidelines in health care. A format for writing clinical practice guidelines at the institutional level is presented in Exhibit 3–2. Mozena, Emerick, and Black (1996) provide instructions for developing algorithms, which depict clinical decision making in a branching format or "decision tree" and are graphic representations of clinical guidelines. Algorithms are very specific, and are particularly useful in the management of high-risk subgroups of patients (Wojner, 1997b).

The difference between critical pathways and clinical pathways is of particular interest. *Critical pathways* specify key elements of care that must be provided—those interventions that are critical to patient care because they have been proven, through scientific inquiry, to influence outcomes. *Clinical pathways* include all elements of care, without specific regard to proven outcomes. Critical pathways have been used primarily in critical care areas in hospitals. Several excellent resources for information about critical pathways include (Hoffman, 1993; Kaine, 1992; Zander, 1993).

A typical clinical pathway is structured so that the categories, types, and sequencing of interventions form the *x* axis, and the timing of treatments (usually day-by-day or week-by-week in some care settings) form the *y* axis. At first, pathways did not include expected intermediate outcomes of care, but work by Karen Zander (1995) and others at the Center for Case Management in South Natick, Massachusetts, produced a second generation of pathways called CareMaps® that compare sets of interventions to sets of intermediate outcomes along the timeline. A sample multidisciplinary clinical pathway format, including space for stating desired patient outcomes, is presented in Exhibit 3–3.

Exhibit 3–1 Clinical Practice Documents

Clinical Practice Guidelines	Multidimensional Clinical Pathways	Preprinted Orders/ Order Sets	Supportive Documentation Tools
Practice guidelines are specifications for medical care developed by a format process that incorporates the best scientific evidence of effectiveness with expert opinion. Practice guidelines should be developed by practitioners involved in the care of a given condition and should be based on rigorous clinical research and soundly generated professional consensus. The guidelines are intended to specify recommendations for treatment methods regarding medical diagnosis and procedure. Practice guidelines are unlike standards, which are meant to be rigidly followed in virtually all cases. Algorithm: Algorithms are flow diagrams that consist of branching logic pathways, which permit the application of carefully defined criteria to the task of identifying or classfiying different types of some entity. As a component of the clinical practice guideline, the algorithm is a written guide to stepwise evaluation and management strategies that require observations to be made, decisions to be considered, and actions to be taken. Algorithms are useful formats for describing and organizing the multiple factors and considerations that characterize medical diagnosis and treatments.	A *companion document* to clinical practice guidelines, which provides an optimal sequencing and timing of interventions by physicians, nurses, and other staff for a particular diagnosis or procedure, designed to minimize delays and resource utilization and to maximize quality. The multidimensional clinical pathway creates a matrix that profiles interventions on one axis and time on the other. Critical pathway: A treatment regimen that includes only a few vital elements proven to affect patient outcomes.	A *companion document* to a practice guideline that facilitates implementation of and compliance with guidelines. • Preprinted orders expedite order process, and reduce variation in care. • May include orders to initiate protocol. Protocol: A detailed document specifying the care to be provided to a patient undergoing a particular treatment. Protocols are strict management directives.	A *companion document* that the caregiver uses to document that the guideline was followed and expected outcomes were met (e.g., cued flowsheets, progress notes, etc.). Examples: • cued flowsheets • progress notes • outcomes measurement worksheet

Courtesy of Leadership Council for Value Enhancement, Ohio State University Medical Center, 1996, Columbus, Ohio.

Exhibit 3–2 Clinical Practice Guideline Components

OBJECTIVE

A statement of the objectives or expected outcomes (value) of the guideline. This statement helps to determine outcomes measurements.

GUIDELINE STATEMENT(S)

Brief guideline statement(s), including the strength of the recommendations, based on levels of evidence. The quality of evidence determines the strength of the guideline.

Quality of evidence:

- *Good:* Evidence obtained from at least one properly randomized controlled trial or from well-designed cohort or case-controlled analytic studies, preferably from more than one center or research group, or national consensus panel recommendations based on controlled, randomized studies.
- *Fair:* Evidence obtained from multiple time series with or without intervention, or national consensus panel recommendations based on uncontrolled studies with positive outcomes or based on studies showing dramatic effects of an intervention.
- *Poor:* Opinions of respected authorities, based on clinical experience, descriptive studies, or reports of expert committees.

KEY WORDS

To expedite literature search.

DEFINITIONS

Explain abbreviations, acronyms, or other terminology for clarification and consistent interpretation.

BACKGROUND INFORMATION

- *Purpose of guideline*
- *Importance of issue:* High prevalence, high incidence, high cost, high degree of variation in practice, other. Documentation to verify information may include statistics on prevalence, incidence, cost and/or citations in the research literature regarding conflicting results or existing protocols.
- *Appropriateness:* Provide a citation to document appropriateness, to include recommendations that differentiate between outpatient and inpatient services or preexisting conditions of patients.

continues

Exhibit 3–2 continued

- *Applicability:* Include disclaimers and/or a discussion of the limitation and/or degree of applicability of the recommendations specific to clinical conditions. Provide a citation to document applicability.
- *Patient preference:* If the guideline includes data regarding patient preferences, a citation to document this may include research findings regarding patients' preference of one course of treatment versus another discussed within the guideline. If the guideline defines patient-oriented measures derived from the guideline, a citation to document this may include surveys of patients' satisfaction with the course of treatment recommended within the guideline.

RECOMMENDATIONS

Recommended diagnostic procedures and treatment, specifying the strength of recommendation and the quality of evidence.

ALGORITHM

A flow diagram that conveys the scope of the guideline, showing clinical choices and outcomes for complicated decision-making processes. The algorithm is an essential teaching component.

REFERENCES

A list of references used in development of the guideline to support the recommendations.

AUTHOR IDENTIFICATION

Name and department of physician-author.

IMPLEMENTATION PLAN

Guidelines will be made widely available and emphasized as part of the educational mission of the medical center. Implementation plans will be developed in cooperation with the author at the time of guideline approval.

EVALUATION/OUTCOMES MEASUREMENT

Once implemented, improvements in clinical practice will be monitored on a periodic basis. This process will be streamlined to produce the most pertinent data within the capabilities and resources of the medical center.

continues

Exhibit 3–2 continued

Measurement includes definition by the guideline author of four "key clinical indicators":

- two process indicators (e.g., the completion of a test/procedure, the prescribing of a medication or therapy that is recommended by the guideline)
- Two outcomes indicators, from one of the four categories of the outcomes measurements compass:
  1. patient satisfaction
  2. clinical outcome
  3. functional outcome
  4. cost

NOTE

Practice guidelines are not standards that are meant to be applied rigidly and followed in virtually all cases. Patient choice and physician judgment must remain central to the selection of diagnostic tests and therapy. Practice guidelines should be helpful to physicians and patients alike in making their decisions.

Courtesy of Ohio State University Medical Center, 1998, Columbus, Ohio.

An approach to mapping rehabilitation care was presented by Court, Loupus, and Morrison (1998) of Shepherd Center, Inc., in Atlanta, Georgia. The CarePath© is the plan of care, the team conference report format, and the primary documentation tool. A charting-by-exception model is used. According to these authors, "Staff are now able to focus their energies on creating new solutions for problems that require individualization, while ensuring that the core plan of treatment is not forgotten" (p. 45). Clinical intervention categories include health status, mobility, activities of daily living, psychosocial, education, community reintegration, and discharge planning. Unlike traditional day-to-day pathways, CarePaths are organized according to the following phases of care: evaluation stage (admission to 72 hours); acute phase (specific criteria are used to classify medically unstable patients who are not ready for intensive rehabilitation); and various rehabilitation phases which, although organized by week, depend upon the patient's achievement of key goals for advancement.

Staff members at Cox Medical Systems of Springfield, Missouri, also use a rehabilitation phase system in their CarePath. Their pathway document, which includes functional status ratings, assessment results, a team conference format, team interventions, and a discharge summary, serves as

Exhibit 3–3 Multidisciplinary Clinical Pathway: Sample Format

Key for desired patient outcomes:
M = Met
NM = Not met

Exclusions if any: ____________
Expected LOS: ____________
Approval date: ____________

	Pre-Admission Date: ________	Time	M/NM	Initial	Hospital Day #1 Date: ________	Time	N/NM	Initial
Desired patient outcome/status								
Care site (may include admission, transfer, and discharge criteria)								
Assessments (may include cardiac, gastro-intestinal, genitourinary, integumentary, musculo-skeletal, neurological, peripheral vascular/circulation, pain, psycho-social/coping, diet/appetite, wound/incision, etc.)								
Consults/tests								
Medications/IV therapy								
Nutrition								
Activity								
Other treatments/interventions (may include consents, respiratory therapy, physical therapy, wound care, etc.)								
Teaching								
Discharge planning/psychological intervention								

Signature Title Initial   *Signature Title Initial*   *Signature Title Initial*

Signature Title Initial   *Signature Title Initial*   *Signature Title Initial*

Signature Title Initial   *Signature Title Initial*   *Signature Title Initial*

Note: This pathway is a general guideline. Patient care continues to require individualization based on patient needs and responses.
Courtesy of Ohio State University Medical Center, 1997, Columbus, Ohio.

both a tracking tool to accompany treatment guidelines and the patient's medical record. The skills acquisition phase of the Cox Medical System's CarePath for cerebrovascular accident rehabilitation is presented in Exhibit 3–4. The term *functional standard* refers to the facility-developed, profession-specific guidelines for intervention, which correspond to functional assessment levels (such as maximum assistance needed, modified independence, supervision level of care).

Cox Medical Systems uses both interdisciplinary and profession-specific treatment guidelines to accompany the CarePath document. These guidelines, which many would call the actual pathway, correspond to the categories listed in the CarePath. The guidelines specify what interventions should be provided, and the expected process (or intermediate)

Exhibit 3–4 CarePath for Cerebrovascular Accident Rehabilitation: Skills Acquisition Phase

__Right __ Left Hemiparesis	Patient: Date:
	PATIENT RESPONSE
Precautions	**SWALLOWING** Functional standard _______ Coughing episodes _______ Verbal cues _______ Equipment _______
Medical	**MEDICAL** **NUTRITION**
Discharge Planning	**INVOLVED CAREGIVER**
Self-Care	**EATING** Functional Standard ________ Hand utilized ________ Physical assist ________ Equipment ________ Verbal cues ____ **GROOMING** Functional standard ______ Hand utilized ______ Physical assist _______ Equipment _____ Verbal cues _____Location ______ **BATHING** Functional standard ______ Hand utilized _____ Physical assist ______ Equipment _____ Verbal cues _____ Location _______ **DRESSING—UPPER EXTREMITY** Functional standard ______ Hand utilized ______ Physical assist ______ Equipment ____ Verbal cues ______ Location ____ **DRESSING—LOWER EXTREMITY** Functional standard _______ Hand utilized _____ Physical assist _____ Equipment _____ Verbal cues _____ Location ____ **TOILETING** Functional standard _______ Hand utilized _______ Physical assist _____ Equipment ______ Verbal cues ____ Location ___ **SELF MEDICATION** Functional Standard ____________ **BOWEL** Functional standard ______ # of accidents _____ Physical assist _____ Equipment _____ Verbal cues _____ Location _____ **BLADDER** Functional standard ______ # of accidents _____ Physical assist ______ Equipment _____ Verbal cues ____ Location_______

continues

Exhibit 3–4 continued

Acuity/Mobility	**WHEELCHAIR MOBILITY** Functional standard _____ Distance _____ Method _____ Physical assist _____ Verbal cues ____
	TRANSFERS Functional standard _____ Type _____ Physical assist _____ Equipment _____ Direction (R,L, both) _____ Verbal cues _____
	TOILET TRANSFERS Location __________ Functional standard _____ Type _____ Physical assist _____ Equipment _____ Direction (R,L, both) _____ Verbal cues _____
	TUB/SHOWER TRANSFER Location __________ Functional standard _____ Type _____ Physical assist _____ Equipment _____ Direction (R,L, both) ____ Verbal cues _____
	GAIT Functional standard _____ Distance _____ Method _____ Equipment _____ Physical assist _____ Verbal cues ____
	STAIRS Functional standard _____ Steps _____ Equipment _____ Physical assist _____ Verbal cues _____
Cognition/Communication	**COMPREHENSION** Functional standard _______________
	EXPRESSION Functional standard _______________
	PROBLEM SOLVING Functional standard _______________
	ATTENTION Functional standard _______________
	MEMORY Functional standard _______________
	LEISURE Functional Standard _______________
Psychosocial Adjustment	**FAMILY ADJUSTMENT** Functional standard __________ **PATIENT ADJUSTMENTS** Functional standard ____________ **SOCIAL INTERACTION** Functional standard __________ Patient ____ Family ____ Pt/Family ____ Time of intervention _____

Courtesy of Cox Rehabilitation Services, Cox Health Systems, 1998, Springfield, Missouri.

outcomes according to phases of care (assessment, treatment, and discharge). The organization's interdisciplinary treatment guidelines for addressing patients' problem-solving skills in the inpatient rehabilitation setting are presented in Exhibit 3–5.

Exhibit 3–5 Interdisciplinary Treatment Guidelines: Inpatient Rehabilitation Problem Solving

Primary responsibility key:

RN-Nursing	SP-Speech pathology
MD-Physician	OT-Occupational therapy
SW-Social services	PT-Physical therapy
PSY-Psychological services	RD-Dietitian
TR-Therapeutic recreation	

Professionals with primary responsibility listed first.

Standards of care

1. Patient will be assessed for functional level of problem solving that promotes participation in the rehabilitation program and safe return home.
2. Patients unable to demonstrate functional problem solving will be provided with recommendations as to need and degree of supervision.
3. Patient and family/caregiver will be counseled regarding need for appropriate discharge plan, including adequate supervision to ensure patient safety.

PROBLEM	ASSESSMENT		TREATMENT		DISCHARGE	
	INTERVENTIONS	PROCESS OUTCOMES	INTERVENTIONS	PROCESS OUTCOMES	INTERVENTIONS	PROCESS OUTCOMES
PRE-MORBID	Assess premorbid function. *All*	1. Assessment completed. 2. Problem list identified. 3. Treatment plan developed based on identified needs.				
MEDICAL/COMPLICATIONS	Assess medications for possible side effects. *MD*					
NUTRITION/HYDRATION						
SELF-CARE	Assess patient's problem-solving skills for: • basic activities of daily living • safety • leisure activities • vocational skills • ambulation/ mobility Consider discharge goals (i.e., independent vs. need for supervision). *SP,OT,PSY,RN,PT*		Provide graded cuing, feedback, modeling to reduce risk and ensure safety. *OT,RN,PT* Monitor patient's functional level of problem solving for reduced injury. *All* Develop problem-solving strategies, identify level of problem solving, trial in functional settings. *OT,SP,PT,RN*	Reduced cues need to ensure safety and participation in rehabilitation program. Equipment/devices recommended. Patient/caregiver demonstrate knowledge to support treatment plan and follow safety recommendations.	Finalize home management techniques for safe home environment and functioning at greater level of independence. *OT,RN,PT*	Safe home environment with supervision as needed.
MOBILITY	Assess patient's problem-solving skills for ambulation/mobility skills. *PT,OT*		Provide graded cues, feedback, modeling for safety during mobility activities. *PT,OT,RN*	Carryover of safety techniques demonstrated in a variety of settings.	Monitor problem-solving skills/safety awareness during community reentry activities. Identify supervision required for discharge. *PT,OT,RN*	Safety techniques finalized in home setting. Caregiver has been educated regarding need for and degree of supervision.

continues

Exhibit 3–5 continued

PROBLEM	ASSESSMENT		TREATMENT		DISCHARGE	
	INTERVENTIONS	PROCESS OUTCOMES	INTERVENTIONS	PROCESS OUTCOMES	INTERVENTIONS	PROCESS OUTCOMES
COGNITION/ COMMUNICATION	Assess verbal problem solving, functional problem solving, and executive functions *SP,PSY*	1. Assessment completed. 2. Problem list identified. 3. Treatment plan developed based on identified needs.	Provide graded cuing, feedback for functional problem-solving situations (verbal and actual). Provide reorientation to promote improved insight. *SP,PSY,OT,PT,RN*	Graded cuing techniques established to promote independence with reduced safety risk. Problem-solving strategies established.	Monitor problem-solving skills/safety awareness during community reentry activities. Identify need for and degree of supervision required at time of discharge. *SP,PSY,OT,PT*	Caregiver/patient demonstrate understanding of discharge recommendations for supervision.
PSYCHOSOCIAL	Assess need for caregiver (full-time, part-time) at discharge. *SW, All*		Work with family to ensure necessary support. *SW,PSY* Identify discharge plan/options/support based on prognosis. *SW*	Caregiver identified, if needed.	Identify community integration issues and make recommendations. *SP,OT,PT,SW*	Appropriate resources provided to ensure patient safety.
EDUCATION	Assess patient knowledge base. *All*		Identify areas for education for patient. *All* Educate patient/caregiver for all new interventions. *All*	Education provided appropriate to identified needs. Education checklist completed for all areas (e.g., devices, equipment, transfer techniques).	Finalize patient and caregiver education as needed. *All* Educate family/patient regarding problem-solving skills. *SP,PSY*	Education completed. Appropriate written materials provided.

Courtesy of Cox Rehabilitation Services, Cox Health Systems, 1998, Springfield, Missouri.

Protocols are the most prescriptive of the structured care methodologies. They specify, in stepwise fashion, what procedures should be performed to accomplish a particular result and ensure that each practitioner who performs the procedure is doing it the same way. Protocols are often developed by individual organizations, but they also appear in national publications (for example, see *Dysphagia Evaluation Protocol* by Avery-Smith, Rosen, and Dellarosa, 1997). A protocol for assessing aspiration pneumonia, which was developed at the Ohio State University Medical Center, is presented in Exhibit 3–6.

The overall purpose of structured care methodologies or clinical decision support tools is to achieve desired patient outcomes by faciliating the effectiveness and efficiency of patient care. Structured care methodologies can also be used for a variety of related reasons, including quality improvement activities, staff orientation, patient and family education, utilization management initiatives, cost-reduction efforts, regulatory compliance, meeting accreditation standards, and marketing to managed care organizations. Kreitner (1994) developed the following list to define clinical pathways:

- the corporate clinical memory
- an antidote to unrestrained clinical variation
- an aid to population-based clinical practice
- systematic precare planning and postcare analysis of variation
- application of sound management science
- the core of a learning process

According to Kreitner (1994), the underlying assumption of structured care is that the systematic study of variation in practice leads to improved clinical processes, followed by improved patient outcomes and reduced resource use. Kreitner emphasizes that clinical pathways are not intended to deter experimentation or innovation, substitute for clinical competence, or generate more paperwork. If some persons have called structured care methodologies "cookbook medicine," they must blame themselves because teams of practitioners have devised the recipes.

Organizations that undertake the important task of developing guidelines, pathways, and other methodologies will likely want to follow these steps recommended by McRury (1998) advice when defining steps in pathway development:

Exhibit 3–6 Protocol for Assessing Aspiration Pneumonia

POLICY

The status of all patients who develop pneumonia and who have received evaluation (bedside or videofluoroscopy) and/or treatment services for dysphagia will be reviewed by the speech-language pathologist (SLP) according to the established protocol. The purpose of the review is to assess the evaluation and treatment services provided by the SLP and to correct any identified problems regarding the patient's ability to swallow safely. The review is conducted in consultation with the medical staff.

PROCEDURE

1. Upon notification that a patient has developed pneumonia, the SLP, with the approval of the physician, will recommend that the patient receive nothing by mouth during the review period.
2. The physician and SLP will determine if the pneumonia has resulted from aspiration, and the SLP will conduct a complete review of the previously established eating plan, if the physician concurs.
3. If the physician determines that the pneumonia is unrelated to aspiration or dysphagia, no further inquiry regarding aspiration will be pursued. SLP consultation will be documented in the progress note section of the medical record.
4. Review of the safe swallowing plan will include:
   - review of the bedside swallowing evaluation and/or videofluoroscopy report (including videotape)
   - ongoing progress reports and medical record entries
   - patient/family reports (interview; observations)
   - review of menu selection with dietitian
   - review of nursing care (interview, nursing notes)
   - review of respiratory care (chart review, interview)
5. The SLP will reevaluate the patient using a bedside swallowing evaluation and/or videofluoroscopy study, as appropriate and approved by the physician.
6. The physician and SLP will discuss the findings of any repeated study and the review of the swallowing plan and agree upon a course of action.
7. The swallowing plan will be reestablished, with modifications as determined by review.
8. The patient, family, and staff will be reeducated about the patient's needs for special diets, feeding techniques, and precautions. Proce-

continues

Exhibit 3–6 continued

dures, results, recommendations, and training will be documented in appropriate records.

FOLLOW-UP PLAN

The SLP will directly monitor the patient's first meal following initiation of the previous or new plan, and two to three times per week thereafter, for a minimum of one week.
The frequency and type of monitoring (e.g., direct observation versus staff report) can be varied, based upon patient need. These are determined weekly.
Monitoring services may later be discontinued per discharge criteria of the Speech Pathology Department dysphagia protocol.
The results of monitoring will be documented.

Courtesy of Rehabilitation Services Division, Ohio State University Medical Center, 1997, Columbus, Ohio.

1. Establish a multidisciplinary team.
   - Include key physicians.
   - Include a representative of each profession or point of service on the pathway.
   - Choose project leaders wisely. Teams may want to have cochairs in addition to a physician sponsor or leader.
2. Decide on a beginning and end point of the care segment along the continuum.
3. Gather baseline data (such as current length of stay, patient satisfaction survey data, outcomes measures, costs, charges, reimbursement).
4. Determine resources available (existing guidelines, protocols, other pathways, benchmark data, evidence in the literature).
5. Identify outcomes to be achieved (patient-focused, measurable, most important to patient progress).
6. Specify level of detail desired in content of document.

Pathways (and other methodologies) must be revised as new scientific and technical information becomes available in order to achieve a best-practice model of care. According to Wojner (1997b), structured care methodologies "should be viewed as dynamic, not static, in that they are never a final product but are in a continuous state of enhancement" (p. 47).

Other indications for revision of structured care methodologies include identification of unnecessary pathway elements, consistent achievement of better-than-expected outcomes, lack of change in patient outcomes, a change in resources, or a change in payer policies (McRury, 1998).

THE AMERICAN SPEECH-LANGUAGE-HEARING ASSOCIATION'S CONTINUUM OF PRACTICE DOCUMENTS

ASHA has provided a continuum of practice documents for speech-language pathologists and audiologists who seek guidance in approaching patient/client services. The purpose of these documents is to enhance the quality of professional services. The ASHA "Code of Ethics" serves as the overall guide for practice. The scope and content of the documents range from broad and general (scope of practice) to narrow and detailed (practice guidelines). Scope of practice statements for audiology (ASHA, 1996a) and speech-language pathology (ASHA, 1996b) provide a list of professional activities that define each profession's range of services. The categories of preferred practice patterns (ASHA, 1997b), position statements, and practice guidelines are defined here as follows:

- *preferred practice patterns*—statements that define universally applicable characteristics of activities directed toward individual patients/clients, and that address structural requisites of the practice, processes to be carried out, and expected outcomes
- *position statements*—statements that specify ASHA's policy and stance on a matter that is important not only to the membership but also to other outside agencies or groups
- *practice guidelines*—a recommended set of procedures for a specific area of practice, based on research findings and current practice, that details the knowledge, skills, and/or competencies needed to perform the procedures effectively

According to ASHA (1997b), the preferred practice patterns "provide an informational base to promote delivery of quality patient/client care. They are sufficiently flexible to permit both innovation and acceptable practice variation, yet sufficiently definitive to guide practitioners in decision-making for appropriate clinical outcomes" (p. 6). ASHA (1997b) provides detailed information about the preferred practice patterns. Information about position statements and practice guidelines can be found in the current version of the *ASHA Desk Reference* (ASHA, 1997a).

DISEASE MANAGEMENT AND DEMAND MANAGEMENT: NEW APPLICATIONS FOR STRUCTURED CARE METHODOLOGIES

Until recently, structured care methodologies have most often been used in inpatient settings, and have been focused on episodes of care. Managed care's emphasis on planning, controlling, and coordinating health care services across time and care settings for defined populations has expanded the use of structured care methodologies within a disease management model. According to Harvey and DePue (1997a, p. 36), disease management "promotes the timely application of proven interventions to prevent healthy populations from becoming ill, ill populations from becoming chronically ill, and chronically ill populations from becoming catastrophically ill." Disease management involves a comprehensive, integrated approach across the entire care continuum so that resources are used in the most cost-effective manner. The focus is on total case costs and long-term outcomes for a targeted population. According to Forer (1998), the core components of a disease management program are risk assessment, environmental assessment, case management, demand management, use of clinical guidelines/algorithms and pathways, patient and care provider education, outcomes tracking, and behavior modification of the target population.

Disease management programs typically focus on populations that are likely to consume the greatest portion of health care resources. Examples of high-risk diagnoses include acquired immune deficiency syndrome (AIDS), arthritis, asthma, brain injury, congestive heart failure, diabetes, heart disease, osteoporosis, and spinal cord injury. The point of disease management programs for these populations is to determine what interventions, programs, medications, and materials offered across the continuum of care will achieve optimal outcomes at the least cost. Structured care methodologies are an important component of disease management programs because they increase coordination of care and flow of information among providers, and provide a guide to or map of the agreed-upon procedures or services. In the disease management model, structured care methodologies are recast to span the entire continuum, incorporating disease staging, risk appraisal, and patient segmentation (Harvey & DePue, 1997b).

Demand management can be part of disease management programs, when focused on specific diagnostic populations, or as part of overall managed care activities for relatively healthy enrollees. As part of disease management programs, demand management is a strategy to reduce high-cost hospital and practitioner use among high-risk groups. Outpatient care, self-management, medication monitoring, behavior modification programs, education, and various levels of prevention activities are emphasized. Sterneck (1997) discusses a number of studies that support the success of demand management in reducing costs while placing patients in the appropriate level of care. Marosits (1997) contends that successful demand management programs "enhance both health outcomes and financial performance through delivery of appropriate services, increased personalization of health management, and risk factor reduction" (p. 44).

According to Marosits (1997), demand management as a managed care strategy has evolved from early models that curtailed costs through financial incentives for physicians (such as fee withholding and capitation) and disincentives for patients (such as using primary care physicians as gatekeepers, copayments, visit limits, exclusions) to models that include clinically focused strategies. Structured care methodologies (or clinical decision support tools) provide the support to match individuals with the most appropriate services. Jacobs (1997) reports that tools such as practice guidelines help manage demand rationally and minimize concerns about over- and underutilization of services because care decisions are based upon explicit, impartial referents. Other uses of clinical decision support tools in demand management include screening proposed interventions for medical appropriateness, determining the most appropriate interventions for a given case, and measuring clinical performance and outcomes by providing best-practice benchmarks. Jacobs (1997) summarizes demand management succinctly: "Coupling patient-specific, clinical decision support tools available at the point of care with the prevailing institution or network system of utilization management can help providers decrease unnecessary demand for resources and justify the use of necessary resources, thus balancing financial and administrative controls with clinically informed guidance" (p. 42).

CONCLUSION

Speech-language pathologists can play an important part in developing structured care methodologies on national, state, and local levels. Members of the profession should ensure their inclusion on development teams for all types of clinical decision-making documents. Furthermore, speech-language pathologists would be wise to initiate profession-specific protocols as part of standard and special order sets. Collaboration with physicians and other professionals will increase speech-language pathologists' visibility and demonstrate their commitment to efficiency, cost reduction, and care based upon sound evidence of effectiveness. Such work is an integral part of clinical practice management and advocacy for speech-language pathologists' services, now and in the future.

Discussion Questions

1. What is clinical accountability and how is it related to the use of structured care methodologies?
2. How are outcomes management principles incorporated into the use of clinical pathways?
3. Why are structured care methodologies used as case management tools?
4. How might speech-language pathologists ensure the inclusion of their services in hospital settings?
5. How are speech-language pathologists involved in disease management?

REFERENCES

Agency for Health Care Policy and Research (1995a). *Using clinical practice guidelines to evaluate quality of care: Vol. 1.: Issues* (AHCPR Publication 95–0045). Rockville, MD: U.S. Department of Health and Human Services.

Agency for Health Care Policy and Research (1995b). *Using clinical practice guidelines to evaluate quality of care: Vol. 2. Methods* (AHCPR Publication 95–0046). Rockville, MD: U.S. Department of Health and Human Services.

Agency for Health Care Policy and Research. (1997, July). AHCPR news and notes. *AHCPR Research Activities, 206*, 13–14.

American Speech-Language-Hearing Association. (1994). Code of ethics. *Asha, 36* (Suppl. 13), 1–2.

American Speech-Language-Hearing Association. (1996a). Scope of practice in audiology. *Asha, 38* (Suppl. 16), 12–15.

American Speech-Language-Hearing Association. (1996b). Scope of practice in speech-language pathology. *Asha, 38* (Suppl. 16), 16–20.

American Speech-Language-Hearing Association. (1997a). *ASHA desk reference.* Rockville, MD: Author.

American Speech-Language-Hearing Association. (1997b). *Preferred practice patterns for the profession of speech-language pathology.* Rockville, MD: Author.

Avery-Smith, W., Rosen, A., & Dellarosa, D. (1997). *Dysphagia evaluation protocol.* San Antonio, TX: Therapy Skill Builders.

Cornett, B., & Chabon, S. (1988). *The clinical practice of speech-language pathology.* Columbus, OH: Merrill.

Court, D., Loupus, D., & Morrison, S. (1998). CarePaths: A tool for coping with managed care. *Topics in Spinal Cord Injury Rehabilitation, 3* (4), 44–52.

Domholdt, E. (1997). Guided by evidence: Assessing similarity of your patients and outcomes to those described in studies. *PT Magazine, 5* (10), 59–65.

Douglass, R. (1983). Defining and describing clinical accountability. *Seminars in Speech and Language, 4* (2), 107–118.

Ellwood, P. (1988). Outcomes management: A technology of patient experience. *New England Journal of Medicine, 318*, 1549–1556.

Field, M., & Lohr, K. (Eds.). (1992). *Guidelines for clinical practice.* Washington, DC: National Academy Press.

Forer, S. (1998). Outcomes and case management. *Rehab Management, 6* (3), 92–95.

Frattali, C. (1998). Quality improvement. In C. Frattali (Ed.), *Measuring outcomes in speech-language pathology* (pp. 172–185). New York: Thieme Medical Publishers.

Frattali, C., & Cornett, B. (1994). Improving quality in the context of managed care. In Ad Hoc Committee on Managed Care (Eds.), *Managing managed care* (pp. 33–42). Rockville, MD: American Speech-Language-Hearing Association.

Harvey, N., & DePue, D. (1997a, June). Disease management: A continuum approach. *Healthcare Financial Management*, 35–37.

Harvey, N., & DePue, D. (1997b, June). Disease management: Program design, development, and implementation. *Healthcare Financial Management*, 38–42.

Hoffman, P. (1993). Critical path method: An important tool for coordinating care. *Journal on Quality Improvement, 19*, 235–246.

Jacobs, C. (1997, July). Managing demand using clinical decision support tools. *Healthcare Financial Management*, 41–43.

Joint Commission on Accreditation of Healthcare Organizations. (1998, September 22). *Improving patient care using case management, clinical pathways, and practice guidelines: Examples of compliance* (Joint Commission Videoconference Series). Oakbrook Terrace, IL: Author.

Kamhi, A. (1984). Problem solving in child language disorders: The clinician as clinical scientist. *Language, Speech and Hearing Services in the Schools, 15* (4), 226–234.

Kaine, R. (1992). Practice protocols by a different name are not quite the same. *Hospital Rehab, 2*, 124.

Kreb, R., & Wolf, K. (1997). *Successful operations in the treatment-outcomes-driven world of managed care.* Rockville, MD: National Student Speech-Language-Hearing Association.

Kreitner, C. (1994, October 1). *Developing critical paths in patient care.* Paper presented at Rehab Expo, Ft. Lauderdale, FL.

Levenson, S. (1996). *Subacute and transitional care handbook.* St. Louis, MO: Beverly-Cracom.

Mahn, V., & Heller, C. (1994). Clinical paths at Carondelet St. Joseph's Hospital. In P. Spath (Ed.), *Clinical paths: Tools for outcomes management* (pp. 191–214) . Chicago: American Hospital Publishing.

Marosits, M. (1997, August). Improving financial and patient outcomes: The future of demand management. *Healthcare Financial Management,* 43–44.

McDermott, M., & Toerge, J. (1994). *Developing critical paths of rehabilitation care: An instruction manual.* Washington, DC: National Rehabilitation Hospital.

McLaughlin, C., & Kaluzny, A. (Eds.). (1994). *Continuous quality improvement in health care.* Gaithersburg, MD: Aspen Publishers, Inc.

McRury, M. (1998). *Clinical pathways: A quality improvement initiative* [unpublished document]. Columbus, OH: The Ohio State University Medical Center.

Merry, M. (1995). Guidelines and pathways: Where do they fit in? *Inside Case Management, 2* (8), 1–3.

Mozena, J., Emerick, C., & Black, S. (1996). *Clinical guideline development: An algorithm approach.* Gaithersburg, MD: Aspen Publishers, Inc.

O'Neil, E. (1998, Summer). Managing to care. *Front & Center, 2* (4), 2.

Ray, J. (1998). Rehabilitation facility-based case management in evolution: Responding to managed care. *Topics in Spinal Cord Injury Rehabilitation, 3* (4), 36–43.

Shekim, L. (1994, Fall). Critical pathways. *Issue of Quality Improvement Digest.* Rockville, MD: The American Speech-Language-Hearing Association.

Spath, P. (Ed.). (1994). *Clinical paths: Tools for outcomes management.* Chicago: American Hospital Publishing.

Spath, P. (1995). Path-based patient care should build quality into the process. *Journal for Healthcare Quality, 17* (6), 26–29.

Stason, W. (1997). Can clinical practice guidelines increase the effectiveness and cost-effectiveness of poststroke rehabilitation? *Topics in Stroke Rehabilitation, 4* (3), 1–16.

Sterneck, J. (1997, December). Demand management: the other side of the health care reform equation. *PT Magazine, 5* (12), 24–27.

Wojner, A. (1997a, March–April). Widening the scope: From case management to outcomes management. *The Case Manager, 8* (2), 77–82.

Wojner, A. (1997b). Outcomes management: From theory to practice. *Journal of Rehabilitation Outcomes Measurement, 1* (5), 42–54.

Zander, K. (1993). Critical pathways. In M. Melum & M. Finioris (Eds.), *Total quality management: The health care pioneers* (pp. 305–314). Chicago: American Hospital Publishing.

Zander, K. (1995). *Managing outcomes through collaborative care: The application of care-mapping and case management*. Chicago: American Hospital Publishing.

SUGGESTED READINGS

American Health Consultants (1995). *The hospital's critical path manual*. Atlanta: Author.

Kreb, R., & Wolf, K. (1997). *Successful operations in the treatment-outcomes-driven world of managed care*. Rockville, MD: The American-Speech-Language-Hearing Association.

Mozena, J., Emerick, C., & Black, S. (1996). *Clinical guideline development: An algorithm approach*. Gaithersburg, MD: Aspen.

Spath, P. (Ed.) (1997). Beyond clinical paths: Advanced tools for outcomes management. Chicago: American Hospital Publishing.

PART II

Perspectives on Functionality

The concept of "functional" communication is not new, but the managed health care environment and school reform issues have renewed practitioners' interest in demonstrating that speech-language pathology services help patients communicate successfully as they participate in daily life activities. Aten (1994) says that functional treatment refers to a holistic approach that addresses linguistic, cognitive, behavioral, social, and familial factors. Aten defines functional communication individually and considers the "severity of the communication disorder, the premorbid and present self-chosen lifestyle of the patient, and the setting in which that person will ultimately reside" (p. 292).

Nelson (1996) offered the following four key questions to guide speech-language assessment and intervention services, as part of her recommendations for providing curriculum-based language intervention.

1. What does the context require?
2. What does the individual currently do in it?
3. What might the individual do differently to increase success in the future?
4. How might the context be modified to increase success? (p. 18)

Although these questions are intended for school settings, they can be applied to any effort to incorporate principles of functionality in daily clinical practice.

The proposed revision of the World Health Organization's *International Classification of Impairments, Disabilities, and Handicaps (ICIDH)* (WHO, 1980) is titled the *International Classification of Impairments, Activities, and Participation (ICIDH-2)*. The concepts presented in this revision are integral to the current discussion about the importance of considering multiple factors in achieving successful communication outcomes. According to Lux (1998), in the context of a health condition, *activity* (formerly disability) refers to the nature and extent of functioning at the level of the person. The ICIDH-2 examines both abilities and limitations relative to the full range of human activities. *Participation* (formerly handicap) refers to the nature and extent of a person's involvement in life situations. The ICIDH-2 identifies degrees of a person's participation in numerous aspects of social life. The revised classification system is based on a biopsychosocial model in which disablement and functioning are viewed as outcomes of complex, bidirectional, dynamic interactions between health conditions and contextual factors. Lux (1998) relates that one of the purposes of the ICIDH-2 is to "characterize physical, mental, social, economic, or environmental interventions that will improve lives and levels of human functioning" (p. 8).

Lux's view supports the purpose of Part II of this book—to help speech-language pathologists provide services that will improve everyday lives. This section does not address every communication diagnosis or situation that practitioners face but presents models of care, specific suggestions for treatment, and case examples associated with attaining functional (practical) goals. Perhaps Nelson (1996) has said it best: "Effective clinical practices result in changes desired by clients and those who are close to them" (p. 11). After all, the purpose of speech-language pathology services is not to "fix deficits," but to assist individuals to meet their needs.

REFERENCES

Aten, J. (1994). Functional communication treatment. In R. Chapey (Ed.), *Language intervention strategies in adult aphasia* (pp. 292–303). Baltimore: Williams & Wilkins.

Lux, J. (1998, October). Towards a common language for functioning and disablement: ICIDH-2 (the international classification of impairments, activities, and participation). *American Speech-Language- Hearing Association Special Interest Division 11: Administration and Supervision Newsletter, 8* (2), 7–8.

Nelson, N. (1996). Seven habits of highly effective change agents (with apologies to Stephen Covey): Focusing on the needs of school-age students. *Hearsay, Journal of the Ohio Speech & Hearing Association, 1*, 11–25.

World Health Organization (1980). *The international classification of impairments, disabilities, and handicaps (ICIDH).* Geneva, Switzerland: Author.

World Health Organization (1998). ICIDH-2. International classification of impairments, activities, and participation. A manual of dimensions of disablement and functioning. Geneva, Switzerland: Author.

CHAPTER 4

Functional Outcomes and Dysphagia Management

Nancy Swigert

Objectives

- Explain the difference between information obtained in a bedside screening and information obtained from instrumental assessment of swallowing function.
- Describe how rating scales can be used to quantify swallowing impairment.
- Explain how functional outcomes measures are used.
- Establish long-term and short-term goals that are written in functional terms.

INTRODUCTION

Dysphagia management is a challenging area of practice for experienced clinicians as well as for new clinicians. The interrelationships among the anatomy and physiology, neurological innervation, overall medical status of the patient, motivation level, and premorbid status combine to challenge the clinician to make an accurate diagnosis, provide a prognosis, and develop an appropriate treatment plan to achieve the best outcome for the patient.

Dysphagia can result from stroke, traumatic brain injury, head and neck cancer, and other causes of congenital or acquired neurological or physical impairment affecting oral-pharyngeal function. The complications from dysphagia can be severe, and may include dehydration, malnutrition, aspiration pneumonia, and death (Terry & Fuller, 1989; Loughlin, 1989;

Lugger, 1994). Current research indicates that 10% of the hospitalized elderly, 30% of patients in nursing homes, and 25% to 45% of all stroke patients present with swallowing disorders (Lugger, 1994; Gordon, Hewer, & Weda, 1987).

Dysphagia is one of the areas of practice in which it is very easy for speech-language pathologists to maintain a focus on function. Patients and their families help practitioners do this. When a speech-language pathologist enters a patient's room for the first time to perform a bedside/clinical dysphagia evaluation of a patient with a new stroke, it is highly unlikely that the patient's spouse will ask "Will my husband's labial and lingual function improve as a result of treatment?" Family members are going to ask practical questions such as "Will my husband be able to eat and have this tube removed from his nose as a result of your treatment?"

It is important that speech-language pathologists' management of patients with dysphagia focus on the functional outcome. Unfortunately, practitioner's documentation does not always reflect that focus. Consider the following discharge notes:

> Mr. _______ has been seen for therapy 5 times per week for 6 weeks. He now exhibits fair to good lip closure and improved lingual skills, including ability to lift tongue tip to roof of mouth and to produce a forceful *k* sound. This is a significant improvement. In addition, patient's voice is no longer perceived as breathy.

Upon reading such a discharge summary, a medical reviewer might be inclined to ask "So what? What difference did this make to the patient's everyday life?"

A functional discharge summary on the same patient might say the following:

> Mr. _______ has been seen for individual therapy 5 times per week for 6 weeks. At the beginning of treatment he had a nasogastric (NG) tube in place for nutrition and was able to take only small amounts of thickened liquids and pureed textures. His ability to close his lips and move his tongue has improved so much that he can now chew soft foods. His laryngeal closure has improved so that he now has adequate airway protection and can

take thin liquids safely. He no longer needs the nasogastic tube, and takes all nutrition and hydration by mouth.

The same medical reviewer would now be likely to state "What an improvement in this patient's life!" Although improving labial, lingual, and laryngeal movement is a positive outcome, moving from an nasogastric tube and small amounts of thickened liquid to eating and drinking a nearly normal diet is a positive *functional* outcome.

This chapter addresses the following major components of dysphagia management:

- bedside/clinical evaluation
- instrumental assessment of swallowing
- use of functional outcome measures
- setting goals
- determining discharge criteria
- ethical issues
- improving medical outcomes

BEDSIDE/CLINICAL EVALUATION

The bedside/clinical evaluation is more appropriately termed a *bedside screening*. Although the clinical evaluation provides important information, it also has significant limitations. It is not possible with a clinical evaluation to determine the presence of or rule out the possibility of aspiration. Splaingard, Hutchins, Sulton, and Chaudhuri (1988) compared videofluoroscopy with bedside clinical evaluations in the diagnosis of aspiration. Bedside evaluation identified only 42% of these patients. Garon, Engle, & Ormiston (1996) studied 1,000 patients and found that 52% were silent aspirators.

A clinical evaluation is usually the first step in a complete assessment of patients with dysphagia. This bedside evaluation does allow the speech-language pathologist to complete a very functional evaluation of the patient's ability to self-feed and of his or her oral phase skills. Essential components of the bedside/clinical evaluation are presented in the following pages.

Obtaining Appropriate Background Information

Determine the patient's current method of nutrition/hydration and whether he or she is taking a diet by mouth. Also determine how long the patient has had the swallowing problem. Look for subtle signs, such as a family member reporting that the patient has stopped drinking coffee in the morning or no longer eats meat.

Young and Durant-Jones (1997) developed a clinical interview questionnaire that can help determine if problems are concentrated in the areas of physical, social, psychological, or dietary concerns. The questionnaire may be most helpful when the patient has had a gradual onset of dysphagia, but can yield information about sudden onset dysphagia. The questionnaire is presented in Exhibit 4–1.

If the speech-language pathologist uses a team approach, an occupational therapist will more completely assess the patient's eye-hand coordination, visual perception, impulsiveness, hand-to-mouth movement, and fine-motor skills. When the speech-language pathologist does not work closely with an occupational therapist during the evaluation, he or she should observe these skills and refer to an occupational therapist if a more complete assessment is needed. Although clinicians may want to control the initial presentation of liquid and food to the patient during the assessment, it is crucial that the patient attempt to self-feed, so that you can assess potential problems that may compromise safety.

Oral Motor Evaluation

Certainly an evaluation of the patient's oral motor skills is important, but looking at these skills in isolation will not necessarily provide information about how the patient can use these same structures for forming and manipulating a bolus.

Assessment of Swallowing

It is helpful to have a tray of food that contains a variety of textures, flavors, temperatures, and types of liquid to assess swallowing at bedside. A bedside evaluation form (see Exhibit 4–2) can help record observations of the patient's skills with a variety of foods and liquids (Swigert, 1996, p.

Exhibit 4–1 Clinical Interview Questionnaire

INSTRUCTIONS

The patient should be asked to respond with YES if the problem occurs most of the time and NO if it never occurs *or* rarely occurs. The number of YES responses at the end of each section can be used to determine if problems are concentrated in the areas of physical, social, psychological, or dietary concerns. For example, patients may report minor physical problems but show elevated responses on social and psychological concerns.

PHYSICAL CONCERNS

1.	Do you have problems swallowing?	Y	N
2.	Do you have difficulty with your own secretions?	Y	N
3.	Do you ever feel food gets stuck in your throat?	Y	N
4.	Do you cough or choke while eating?	Y	N
5.	Do you need to swallow more than once for each bite?	Y	N
6.	Do you need to chew longer in order to swallow?	Y	N
7.	Do you have difficulty swallowing pills?	Y	N
8.	Do you have pain while swallowing?	Y	N
9.	Does your voice change during or after eating?	Y	N
10.	Do you have nasal regurgitation?	Y	N
11.	Do you have frequent upper-respiratory infections or pneumonia?	Y	N
12.	Do you know of any recent weight loss?	Y	N
	Total:		

SOCIAL CONCERNS

1.	Do you prefer to eat alone?	Y	N
2.	Do you avoid eating with others?	Y	N
3.	Have you stopped eating in restaurants?	Y	N
	Total:		

PSYCHOLOGICAL CONCERNS

1.	Do you feel unsatisfied after eating?	Y	N
2.	Are you afraid of choking?	Y	N
3.	Do you ever feel like not eating?	Y	N
4.	Are you embarrassed about eating?	Y	N
5.	Has your enjoyment of food changed?	Y	N

continues

Exhibit 4–1 continued

6. Do you find that you need to concentrate when swallowing to avoid problems? Y N
7. Do you ever feel fatigue during or following a meal? Y N

Total:

DIETARY CONCERNS

1. Do you dislike the type of food you are eating? Y N
2. Do you avoid certain foods? Y N
3. Are there foods you wish you could swallow again? Y N
4. Do you find some foods easier to eat? Y N
5. Are you concerned about your nutrition? Y N
6. Have you decreased the size of the bites or sips you take? Y N
7. Has the amount of time it takes to consume a meal increased? Y N
8. Do you find alternating foods with a drink makes swallowing easier? Y N
9. Do you use dietary supplements such as Ensure? Y N

Total:

TOTAL

Add the total number of YES responses for each section. Analyze the responses in terms of those areas that have been most affected by swallowing changes.

Affected areas (Check the appropriate categories):

_____ Physical
_____ Social
_____ Psychological
_____ Dietary

Source: Reprinted with permission from E.C. Young and L. Durant-Jones, Gradual Onset of Dysphagia: A Study of Patients with Oculopharyngeal Muscular Dystrophy, *Dysphagia*, Vol. 12, pp. 196–201, © 1997, Springer-Verlag New York, Inc.

46). A patient may exhibit what appear to be adequate oral skills when the speech-language pathologist presents small amounts of food on a spoon and look completely different when self-feeding large bites and sips. Consider the following case:

> Mr. Emery is a patient who has a new onset of right-hemisphere cerebrovascular accident (CVA). He has minimal left labial droop. When presented with food per spoon by the speech-language pathologist, he requires a little assistance to obtain tight lip closure on the spoon to remove the food from the spoon. When trying to prepare a bolus with food that requires mastication, he has significant residue in the left cheek but can clear this when external pressure is provided to the cheek and he is given a verbal cue to clear the cheek with his tongue.
>
> However, when the patient is allowed to hold the fork and feed himself, he is not able to put the fork into his mouth. He hits the corner of his mouth with the fork and loses a lot of the food from the fork. He presents the food very quickly, putting three to four bites in his mouth before he even begins to attempt to manipulate the bolus. He exhibits coughing and choking behavior while trying to manipulate the bolus and also taking a drink of liquid.

This valuable information would not have been obtained had the clinician discontinued the clinical evaluation before observing the patient trying to feed himself. It might have been reported that it was safe for the patient to eat with external pressure to the cheek and some lip support. However, after this more complete evaluation, it is clear that the patient needs help controlling his impulsivity (such as verbal cues to take one bite at a time) and not to mix liquids with solids.

Procedures Sometimes Used During Bedside/Clinical Evaluations

Two procedures are sometimes used during bedside/clinical evaluations—the blue dye test and cervical auscultation. Each of these procedures should be used cautiously and viewed with some skepticism, because there is not sufficient information in the literature at this time to support drawing conclusions from the use of either of these procedures. Unfortunately, each is sometimes used as an actual diagnostic procedure when neither should be considered as such.

Blue Dye Test

The Modified Evans Blue Dye Test (MEBDT) is a modified form of the original Evans Blue Dye Test used with tracheotomized patients (Spray,

Exhibit 4–2 Swallowing Evaluation Form

Patient: Fred   Patient # ________

Swallowing

Key		*Compensatory Techniques*
+ skill is adequate	S straw	TS thermal stimulation
— skill is inadequate	SP spoon	CD chin down
N/A not applicable for that texture	C cup	HR head rotation
	CO cut-out cup	BS bolus size
		EP external pressure

Texture		Liquids	Pureed	Eggs	Honey		
Ability to prepare bolus							
Labial closure	+/—	—	—	—	—		
Lingual elevation	+/—	+	+	+	+		
Lingual lateralization	+/—		+	+	+		
Mastication	+/—	N/A	N/A	—			
Ability to manipulate bolus							
Lingual function	+/—	+	+	—	+		
Oral transit time	+/—+	+	+	—	+		

Ability to maintain bolus							
Back of tongue control	+/—	—	+	+	+		
Labial closure	+/—	—	—	—	—		
Cheeks	+/—	— / EP+	— / EP+	— / EP+	— / EP+		
Lingual lateralization	+/—	N/A	+	+	+		
Clears oral cavity in one swallow	+/—	—	—	—			
Number of swallows per bolus	+/—	2	2	2–3	2		
Pharyngeal phase							
Initiate reflex in ___ seconds	+/—						
Laryngeal characteristics							
Vocal quality	+/describe	CD & wet	wet	wet	wet		
Cough/throat clearing	+/—	+	+	+	+		
Elevation of larynx	+/—	+	+	+	+		

Comments ____

____

Courtesy of LinguiSystems, Inc., East Moline, Illinois.

Zuidema, & Cameron, 1976) in which blue food coloring is mixed with 3 to 5 cc of thin liquid and semisolid food. The patient is then suctioned at the tracheostomy for any sign of blue food coloring. Thompson-Henry and Braddock (1995) used the MEBDT with five patients. The test was negative for all five patients they studied; however, Fiberoptic Endoscopic Evaluation of Swallowing (FEES®) or modified barium swallow (MBS) studies conducted 4 to 22 days later revealed aspiration for all five patients. These authors concluded that examiners should exercise caution when using MEBDT as the primary indicator of a patient's swallow function. Logemann (personal communication, January 1996) points out that a significant problem with the technique is the occurrence of false positives. That is, most people aspirate small amounts, especially during sleep. Tippett and Siebens (1996) contend that the Thompson-Henry and Braddock (1995) study was flawed for a number of reasons including unspecified subject selection criteria, unspecified cuff status during the FEES® and MBS studies, and the influence of the time intervals between the MEBDT and the FEES® or the MBS. However, Tippett and Siebens do agree that caution may be warranted and that false negative readings are conceivable when using the MEBDT. Leder (1996) also raised concerns about the methodology of the Thompson-Henry and Braddock study and noted: "A prospective and randomized or consecutive study using an MBS or FEES® for an objective assessment of aspiration immediately followed by an MEBD procedure is needed to demonstrate the efficacy and sensitivity of the MEBD procedure in assessing aspiration" (p. 81). Clearly, further study is necessary to determine the efficacy of the MEBDT. Until such research is available, dysphagia clinicians may best serve their patients by recognizing that the MEBDT has not been validated as a tool to detect aspiration reliably.

Cervical Auscultation

Cervical auscultation involves placing the head of a stethoscope laterally on the thyroid cartilage and listening to the sounds of swallowing. A normal swallow is presumed to follow this sequence:

1. The individual is heard to breathe.
2. Breathing stops, usually in the exhalation phase.
3. A sound (sometimes described as a swish or a clunk) is heard.
4. Breathing is heard again, and it sounds dry and clear.

Proponents of the use of cervical auscultation indicate that they can "hear aspiration." Zenner, Losinski, and Mills (1995) state that aspiration is suspected if a flushing sound of material is heard prior to initiation of the swallow or when wet breath sounds, coughing, or voice distortion is heard after the swallow. The problem with this approach is that there is not good scientific evidence to indicate that this technique predicts aspiration accurately. Zenner, Losinski, and Mills (1995) performed cervical auscultation on 50 patients at bedside who then had a videofluoroscopic examination (mean of 14.5 days later). The authors reported the following levels of agreement between what they "heard" at bedside and what they saw on videofluoroscopy weeks later: pharyngeal delay, 66%; pharyngeal residuals, 42%; and tracheal aspiration, 76%. Obviously, this study is flawed because the same swallows were not assessed with both methods simultaneously. Even these authors state: "At this time, cervical auscultation is an imprecise clinical method for evaluating risks of tracheal aspiration" (p. 30).

Family/Caregiver Education

The bedside clinical evaluation provides an excellent opportunity for teaching the family or caregiver. They can observe the evaluation and see how the clinician performs techniques that are beneficial for the patient. However, having the family try to use the techniques is probably more helpful than having the family simply observe. Although families may feel uncomfortable actually trying the techniques, clinicians should encourage them to do so. It is particularly difficult for families to give verbal reminders to patients who may perceive this as "nagging." Patients are sometimes less willing to follow directives of family members than those of the speech-language pathologist. Practitioners should help the caregiver and patient feel comfortable using compensatory techniques.

INSTRUMENTAL ASSESSMENT OF SWALLOWING

Videofluoroscopy

A thorough assessment of a patient's pharyngeal and esophageal stages of swallowing requires a videofluoroscopic study, or modified barium swallow (MBS) study. One of the drawbacks of such a study is that it is simply a reflection of the patient's skills during a particular moment in time. Patients, especially in the acute stages of their disease, can demonstrate skills that fluctuate widely. Therefore, the results of the MBS study must be interpreted cautiously. In particular, the effects of fatigue may not be easily observed. In addition, the test creates a very unnatural situation in which most presentations are made by the radiologic technologist or the speech-language pathologist. If the patient appears to be swallowing safely with the clinician's presentations, the patient should be allowed to hold the cup or spoon and present to himself; this provides an opportunity to see if he takes much larger sips or throws his head back.

Obtaining Appropriate History

It is essential that a complete and thorough history be obtained when performing the MBS study. Questions such as those provided in Exhibit 4–3 will allow the speech-language pathologist to analyze the patient's symptoms to make a hypothesis about possible etiology of the disorder. For instance, if the patient says that he notices he is coughing immediately after he eats dinner but does not notice it with other meals, the practitioner might question him further and find out that after dinner he lies down on the couch to watch the evening news. This information might lead to the hypothesis that he is experiencing gastroesophageal reflux, which is causing the coughing. One might also hypothesize that the patient has significant residue in valleculae or pyriforms that is dislodged when he lies down.

These questions may also help the speech-language pathologist determine what needs to be done during the study. For example, if the patient's reply to the interview questions indicates that she is having difficulty making herself heard and that her voice sounds very quiet to her, the clinician would probably complete an anterio-posterior view to assess vocal fold movement, symmetry of residue, and other factors.

The MBS study provides information about the patient's anatomy and physiology. The speech-language pathologist must interpret that information and determine what impact these changes in physiology will have on the patient's function. This interpretation and translation into function is especially important when communicating the results to the family. Consider the following two examples, each of which describes the same patient during the same study.

Exhibit 4–3 Swallowing Questionnaire To Provide Additional History

- When did the problems with your swallowing start?
- Did the start of the swallowing problem coincide with any other medical problems?
- When you eat and drink, do you have any episodes of coughing, choking, etc.?
- Does food or drink ever go "down the wrong way"?
- Do you avoid certain foods because they are hard to swallow?
- Do liquids ever come out your nose?
- Do you ever feel that food gets "stuck" in your throat?
- Do you wake up at night coughing or choking?
- Is your swallowing problem intermittent or constant?
- Has your swallowing problem changed over time?
- Has your voice or speech changed?

Courtesy of LinguiSystems, Inc., East Moline, Illinois.

> Mr. Pope has premature movement of the bolus over the back of the tongue but when the bolus hits the valleculae, the pharyngeal swallow triggers within one second. He has very limited laryngeal elevation with significant residue in the valleculae and the pyriform sinuses with penetration into the upper laryngeal vestibule during the swallow and then trace aspiration after the swallow from the penetrated material. He is silent with this aspiration. The aspiration could be eliminated with a tight chin-down technique to provide better airway protection and multiple swallows.

These same findings can be told in functional language that the family will understand:

> Mr. Pope has some trouble controlling the back of his tongue. This probably doesn't surprise you since you can tell how weak his speech sounds are, especially when he tries to produce sounds like *K* or *G*. This weakness at the back of the tongue lets liquid trickle toward the throat before he is really ready to swallow. When you swallow, your larynx, or "voice box," is supposed to lift up high in the neck to get out of the way and close off the airway so that food or liquid goes to the stomach and not into the

lungs. This does not happen with Mr. Pope. Because his voice box does not lift as high as it needs to, a little opening is left that allows liquid to try to go the wrong way. A little actually does go toward his lungs. This puts him at risk for developing pneumonia. We were able to show Mr. Pope a technique that can keep the liquid from going into his lungs. If he puts his chin down onto his chest, it helps move the voice box out of the way so that liquid does not go down into the lungs. If he also remembers to swallow twice, it helps to clear out a lot of residue that remains in a couple of pockets in his throat.

Measuring Change in Videofluoroscopic Studies

It is difficult to determine a successful outcome of a diagnostic procedure. A procedure such as the MBS study allows the speech-language pathologist to make an accurate diagnosis and to establish an appropriate treatment plan. In that way, a successful outcome to treatment follows from the completion of an appropriate evaluation.

Another way to look at change based on the MBS study is to obtain some objective measurements during the study. If the patient has a repeat study later, the measurements can be taken again and a comparison made. Therefore, the clinician is not just guessing whether the patient has made significant improvement from one evaluation to the next. Many patients have repeat MBS studies. At Central Baptist Hospital in Lexington, Kentucky, of the inpatients who received an MBS study during a one-year period, 12% were seen for a repeat study during that hospitalization. Another 9% were seen for a repeat study during another hospitalization. In addition, 11% of outpatients seen for an evaluation had received a prior study. Rating scales used with those patients allowed clinicians to compare performance and change.

Two rating scales exist that help clinicians obtain objective data during the videofluoroscopic study—the Duke University Medical Center "Rating of Radiologic Swallowing Abnormalities" (Horner, Riski, Ovelmen-Levitt, & Nashold, 1992) and the "Penetration-Aspiration Scale" (Rosenbek, Robbins, Roecker, Coyle, & Wood, 1996). The Duke scale is used to rate functional ability and degree of radiologic abnormality. It uses a four-point rating scale (0 = profound, 1 = severe, 2 = moderate, 3 = mild, and 4 = normal) for each of the following major categories: oral-preparatory phase; reflex initiation phase; pharyngeal phase; pharyngeal appearance observed in anterior-posterior projection; aspiration; and pharyngeal-esophageal phase screening (see Table 4–1 and Exhibit 4–4).

Rosenbek and colleagues (1996) developed an eight-point, equal-interval scale to describe penetration and aspiration during videofluoroscopic studies. These scores are determined primarily by the depth to which material enters the airway and whether or not it is expelled (see Exhibit 4–5).

Although these two scales are based on the speech-language pathologist's judgment, they may provide more objective ratings of baseline behavior to help assign a severity rating and to provide a point of comparison for improvement.

Fiberoptic Endoscopic Evaluation of Swallowing FEES®

The Fiberoptic Endoscopic Evaluation of Swallowing (FEES®) uses a flexible nasendoscope, which is passed transnasally until the tip is slightly below the velum in the hypopharynx. The speech-language pathologist can visualize structures in the hypopharynx and the larynx. The procedure includes an anatomic-physiologic assessment of velopharyngeal closure, base of tongue, airway protection and phonation; the evaluator then presents food/liquids dyed green with food coloring and assesses the swallow (Langmore, 1998).

Murray, Langmore, Ginsberg, and Dostie (1996) used the following rating scale to predict which patients were at risk for aspiration based on the location of secretions: 0 = no excess secretions; 1 = secretions in valleculae, pyriforms, lateral channels; 2 = transitional rating (changed from a 1 to a 3 during the observation); 3 = secretions in laryngeal vesti-

Table 4–1 Global Assessment Ratings

Guideline	*Global Rating*
All categories rated a 4	Normal
Asymmetry of pharyngeal bolus transit occurred in isolation	Slight
One or more dimensions rated 3	Mild
One or more dimensions rated 2, *or* If aspiration occurred in the context of otherwise mildly impaired function	Moderate
One or more dimensions rated 1, *or* If aspiration occurred in the context of otherwise moderately impaired function	Severe

Exhibit 4–4 Duke University Medical Center Rating of Radiologic Swallowing Abnormalities

ORAL-PREPARATORY PHASE

0 = *Profound dysfunction:* oral stasis; no material is propelled into the pharynx.
1 = *Severe dysfunction:* effortful oral preparation; dispersion of the bolus along the tongue and into the buccal cavities; significant oral residue after the swallow that is not cleared; extreme slowness and inefficiency in propelling the bolus into the pharynx; no masticatory ability; drooling usually occurs.
2 = *Moderate dysfunction:* slow oral preparation and motility of boluses; mastication very slow but thorough; some residue along the tongue; inefficiency and effort in propelling the bolus into the pharynx; drooling may also occur.
3 = *Mild dysfunction:* mildly slow bolus preparation, but adequate bolus cohesion and motility; mastication slower than normal but thorough; mild lip incompetency with drooling may be present.
4 = *Normal:* Normal control and bolus transit; no oral residue; mastication is brisk and thorough.

REFLEX INITIATION PHASE

0 = *Profound:* absent reflex.
1 = *Severe:* reflex initiated in the lower pharynx (pyriform sinuses) after prolonged pooling.
2 = *Moderate:* reflex initiated in the lower pharynx after brief hesitation.
3 = *Mild:* reflex initiated in the midpharynx (vallecular spaces) after brief hesitation.
4 = *Normal:* reflex initiated at the back or base of the tongue (above the epiglottis); no hesitation in bolus motility from posterior tongue into pharynx.

PHARYNGEAL PHASE

0 = *Profound residue:* reflex is minimal or absent, and the bolus fills the mid- and lower pharynx; suctioning or vigorous pharyngeal gag and cough are required to clear the pharynx.
1 = *Severe residue:* more than half the bolus remains in the pharynx after the swallow; much effort required to clear the residue, possibly requiring sips of liquid barium or water; poor peristalsis typically associated with the following: (a) weak propulsion force of tongue at reflex initiation; (b) visibly reduced laryngeal elevation and epiglottic tilting;

continues

Exhibit 4–4 continued

and/or (c) incomplete midpharyngeal and laryngopharyngeal closure during the swallow.

2 = *Moderate residue:* more than 10% but less than 50% of the bolus remains in the mid- and/or lower pharynx; requires an extra swallow to clear; usually occurs in association with (a–c) above.

3 = *Mild residue:* less than 10% of a small bolus remains in the mid- and/or lower pharynx after the first swallow.

4 = *Normal:* no residue; slight coating only may be present.

PHARYNGEAL APPEARANCE OBSERVED IN ANTERIOR-POSTERIOR PROJECTION

0 = *No pharyngeal transit:* profound residue in the mid- and/or lower pharynx bilaterally; usually seen only when the reflex is absent.

1 = *Severe:* bilateral pharyngeal weakness characterized by moderate or severe residue in the bilateral pharyngeal spaces (midpharynx, lower pharynx, or both); often the pharynx will appear bilaterally patulous, or bilateral pulsion diverticula will be observed.

2 = *Moderate:* pharyngeal hemiplegia characterized by definite asymmetry; pharyngeal motility only on the opposite (the functional) side.

3a = *Mild:* pharyngeal hemiparesis characterized by bilateral pharyngeal transit that is visibly superior on the opposite side, and/or the hemiparetic side may show a pyriform sinus "droop," and/or the hemiparetic side may show hypotonia of the thyrohyoid membrane presenting as a "pulsion diverticulum."

3b = Slight: postural abnormality; pharyngeal asymmetry with no observable anatomic or physiologic basis (e.g., due to torticollis, poor sitting balance, or head deviation due to neglect, distractibility, etc.) (*Note:* When nondysphagic individuals turn or tilt the head to one side, pharyngeal asymmetry is a normal finding, but pharyngeal asymmetry is considered to be abnormal when head and neck postures are involuntary.)

4 = *Normal:* both symmetrical appearance and symmetrical bolus transit; no anatomic or physiologic abnormalities observed.

ASPIRATION

0 = *Profound:* more than trace aspiration, audible or silent; may include repeated instances of aspiration, despite postural or other modifications to prevent aspiration. If the reflex is absent, risk for aspiration is profound and also warrants a rating of 0.

continues

Exhibit 4–4 continued

1 = *Severe:* more than trace aspiration, audible or silent; may include repeated instances of aspiration, despite postural or other modifications to prevent aspiration. ("Trace" refers to less than 10% of the bolus.)
2 = *Moderate: trace silent* aspiration. (No laryngeal cough during aspiration through the larynx is referred to as "silent aspiration.")
3 = *Mild: trace audible* aspiration. (When aspiration occasions a cough, it is referred to as audible aspiration.)
4 = *No aspiration.* (Risk for aspiration may be present, and should be noted relative to other observations.)

PHARYNGEAL-ESOPHAGEAL PHASE SCREENING

0 = *Profound:* absent swallow reflex; no relaxation of the upper esophageal sphincter (UES); no material enters the esophagus.
1 = *Severe:* severe pyriform sinus residue; sporadic or effortful passage of food or liquid into the upper esophagus; definite indication that the UES is failing to relax; usually associated with a severely incomplete swallowing reflex and reduced laryngeal excursion.
2 = *Moderate:* residue is present in the pyriform sinus(es) in equal or greater amount than in the vallecular space(s), suggesting UES dysfunction, potentially secondary to one or more of the following: (a) decreased pharyngeal peristalsis; (b) dyscoordination (mistiming) of pharyngeal peristalsis and cricopharyngeal relaxation (the material is eventually cleared from the pharynx, but repeated swallows are necessary); (c) incomplete relaxation of the upper esophageal sphincter (when larger boluses are administered, the caliber of the UES is diminished and manometry may be indicated); (d) hypotonia of the UES and/or dyscoordination of UES relaxation manifest as reflux from the upper esophagus into the pyriform sinuses after the swallow.
3 = *Mild:* residue is present in the vallecular space(s) primarily; adequate relaxation of the UES, but the evaluation is limited to small boluses only (larger boluses were precluded by the presence of, or risk for, aspiration).
4 = *No aspiration:* normal relaxation of the UES, evaluated using a gulp or large naturalistic swallow(s).

Source: Reprinted with permission from J. Horner et al., Swallowing in Torticollis Before and After Rhizotomy, *Dysphagia*, Vol. 7, No. 3, pp. 117–125, © 1992, Springer-Verlag New York, Inc.

Exhibit 4–5 Eight-Point Penetration-Aspiration Scale

1. Material does not enter the airway.
2. Material enters the airway, remains above the vocal folds, and is ejected from the airway.
3. Material enters the airway, remains above the vocal folds, and is not ejected from the airway.
4. Material enters the airway, contacts the vocal folds, and is ejected from the airway.
5. Material enters the airway, contacts the vocal folds, and is not ejected from the airway.
6. Material enters the airway, passes below the vocal folds, and is ejected into the larynx or out of the airway.
7. Material enters the airway, passes below the vocal folds, and is not ejected from the trachea despite effort.
8. Material enters the airway, passes below the vocal folds, and no effort is made to eject.

Source: Reprinted with permission from J. Rosenbeck et al., A Penetration-Aspiration Scale, *Dysphagia*, Vol. 11, pp. 93–98, © 1996, Springer-Verlag New York, Inc.

bule, not cleared. In their study of 49 subjects, Murray and colleagues found the following: of patients rated 0, 21% aspirated food or liquid; of patients rated 1, 53% aspirated; of patients rated 2, 100% aspirated; of patients rated 3, 100% aspirated. They concluded that excess secretions visualized with FEES® have a high predictive value for aspiration.

At present there are no standardized recommendations regarding competency to perform this procedure. Clinicians who wish to learn should find someone who performs this procedure—another speech-language pathologist or otolaryngologist—who will agree to teach them how to perform the procedure, supervise them through some limited number of procedures (perhaps 10), and then verify competence.

Some speech-language pathologists express concern that the use of FEES® may lead to an expansion of otolaryngologists' role in the diagnosis of dysphagia. One of the effects of managed care is the reduced number of patients who are referred to specialists, such as otolaryngologists. This situation means that such specialists are interested in other practice opportunities. FEES® should be done by a trained and competent speech-language pathologist and should not be turned over to the otolaryngologist, who primarily examines structures and function for phonation. Conversely, speech-language pathologists must not try to diagnose any structural abnormalities found when performing a FEES®. The speech-language pathologist is obliged to refer the patient to an otolaryngologist if any abnormalities are observed. Therefore, the two professionals (the speech-language pathologist and the otolaryngologist) use nasendoscopy for two very different procedures.

Before beginning a program of FEES®, several things must be determined:

- Do state licensure laws allow speech-language pathologists to perform endoscopy as a part of their scope of practice? This may not be clear in state laws because most were written before anyone began using endoscopy to evaluate swallowing.
- What credentialing process does the facility require for speech-language pathologists to perform this technique?

Comparison of Instrumental Techniques

Is one instrumental study preferred over the other? The FEES® provides better direct visualization of the structures (epiglottis, valleculae, pyriform sinuses, vocal cords, arytenoids). It also allows assessment of the pharyngeal phase by presenting only ice chips, or even during saliva swallows. However, because the tip of the scope is completely obliterated during the swallow, one cannot assess what happens during the swallow.

The MBS study or videofluoroscopy provides better visualization of how the structures function and move together during the swallow (such as anterior and superior movement of the hyoid and larynx). It provides a comprehensive view of the oral, pharyngeal, and esophageal phases. Because the entire bolus can be seen, it is easier to judge the amount of aspiration. A better assessment of the effects of compensatory strategies can also be made.

FUNCTIONAL OUTCOME MEASURES

After a bedside and/or instrumental assessment, it is important to document baseline behavior in order to report change or outcome. Baseline information can be obtained in many ways. More traditional approaches ask the speech-language pathologist to record the number of times the patient loses food out of the front of his mouth or the number of coughs.

Information about improved tongue function or lip function is not very meaningful to the patient, the patient's family, health care providers, or payers. These audiences are demanding functional outcomes—the impact that a treatment has on the patient's ability to function in everyday life.

Functional descriptions of swallowing have appeared in the literature for years. Steefel presented a seven-level rating scale in 1981. These levels ranged from *severe* (judged as nonfunctional), in which all nourishment is given by alternate methods, to *moderate* (interferes with function), in which alternate methods may be withdrawn on a trial basis and the patient continues to receive complete supervision until the patient reaches a normal level of functioning.

Comprehensive functional assessment instruments may also contain scales to assess swallowing. The Functional Independence Measure (FIM) (Uniform Data System, 1995) was designed to measure a level of independence in self-care, sphincter control, transfers, locomotion, communication, and social cognition. Each variable within those categories is scored on a 1-to-7 scale. Unfortunately, the FIM's attempt to assess functional change in swallowing is rated on a self-care scale called "Eating." This scale focuses on the use of suitable utensils to bring food to the mouth, chewing, and swallowing but is not specific enough to measure change in swallowing.

The American Speech-Language-Hearing Association (ASHA, 1998) has developed seven-point rating scales of functional ability in a variety of communication areas. These rating scales, called Functional Communication Measures (FCMs), are an integral part of the National Outcomes Measurement System (NOMS) for speech-language pathology and audiology. This national database is designed to collect outcomes information and answer questions such as the following:

- How many sessions does it take to treat particular disorders?
- How much progress do patients with different disorders make in different settings?
- Is there a difference in the amount of progress made when different service delivery models are used?

The swallowing FCM considers dietary levels/restrictions, including the kinds of solid foods and the kinds of liquids the patient can take safely. The scale also describes the kind of cueing required. Level 1, for instance, reflects no functional swallow with the patient receiving all nutrition and hydration through nonoral means. By level 4, the patient is swallowing safely, but usually requires moderate cues to use certain compensatory strategies. The patient at that level may still have significant diet restrictions or require some tube feeding or oral supplements. By the time the patient reaches level 7, the ability to eat independently is not limited by swallow function and swallowing is considered safe and efficient for all consistencies. At this point, the patient uses compensatory strategies without any extra cueing. (The complete Functional Communication Measure for swallowing is available at no charge to subscribers of ASHA's NOMS. For more information, contact the National Center for Treatment Effectiveness in Communication Disorders at ASHA, 301-897–5700, ext. 4265). A patient is rated on the Functional Communication Measure at admission and at discharge. Statements can be made that reflect the amount of functional change the patient has made over the course of treatment. Consider the difference in the following conversations that might take place with the case manager for an insurance company who asks the speech-language pathologist to document if any changes have occurred in the last four weeks. The first conversation is in nonfunctional terms:

> The patient is exhibiting better lip closure and tongue movement. He still has difficulty manipulating foods that do not stay together in a cohesive bolus. He is now able to take syrup-thick rather than honey-thick liquids.

The second conversation is based upon a functional rating:

> Upon admission, the patient was at level 3 on the ASHA NOMS. He had a nasogastric tube because he could eat less than half of his meals; he was safe to eat with moderate cues to put his chin down and swallow twice, but his diet was maximally restricted in that he required a pureed diet and honey-thick liquids. He is now at a level 5. He no longer requires tube feeding and is on a diet of chopped meats, soft vegetables, and syrup-thick liquids.

Although both of these statements reflect change, the latter is easier for a payer to understand.

Patient satisfaction is another measure of successful outcome. Patient satisfaction tools can take many forms, and facilities and institutions often have a particular format they like to use. Questions such as those presented in Exhibit 4–6 might be included on a patient satisfaction questionnaire, which could be given to the patient and/or caregiver at the conclusion of treatment.

SETTING GOALS

After the evaluation is complete, the speech-language pathologist must develop a treatment plan. It is necessary to identify long- and short-term goals.

Long-Term Goals

The long-term goal is what one hopes the patient will accomplish at the conclusion of treatment. This does not necessarily mean conclusion of

---

Exhibit 4–6 Patient Satisfaction Measure

	Strongly Agree	Agree	Neutral	Disagree	Strongly Disagree
My swallowing skills are better because of the treatment I received.					
The speech-language pathologist explained my swallowing problem and the treatment to me in a way that I could easily understand.					
Overall I am satisfied with the services provided.					
If I knew someone else with a swallowing problem I would refer them here for intervention.					

treatment within a particular setting, but conclusion of treatment at the end of the continuum of care for the patient. For instance, if a practitioner sees patients in an acute-care setting for three to four days, it would not be appropriate to establish a long-term goal based on what a patient will accomplish in those few days or even weeks. A long-term goal should be established based on the best information available about what the patient's ultimate outcome will be.

Long-term goals should be written in functional terms such as the following:

- Patient will safely consume ______ diet with _____ liquids without complications such as aspiration pneumonia.
- Patient will be able to eat foods and liquids with more normal consistency.
- Patient's quality of life will be enhanced through eating and drinking small amounts of food and liquid.

If the speech-language pathologist does not think the patient is a candidate for improvement through intervention, the patient's long-term goal may be:

- Nutrition and hydration will be maintained via an alternative method.

It is important to involve the patient and significant others in establishing the long-term goal. The speech-language pathologist should provide the patient and family with information on the prognosis for improvement, with an idea of what the functional status might be at the end of treatment. The practitioner will have to draw upon what data are available concerning the outcome of patients with dysphagia. There are numerous studies demonstrating the effectiveness of specific treatment techniques, but not as many with information to help make a prognostic statement.

A retrospective review of acute inpatients at Central Baptist Hospital in Lexington, Kentucky, demonstrated the effectiveness of intervention. Of the patients evaluated at bedside, 28% received a modified barium swallow (MBS). As a result of the MBS, 33% were found to be safe with oral intake and had their feeding tube removed; 24% were confirmed to be unsafe to eat, and this finding helped to avoid possible complications like aspiration pneumonia. Of the patients who received dysphagia treatment, 58% showed complete resolution of their dysphagia by discharge.

ASHA's NOMS will eventually accumulate enough data to answer questions such as the following:

- For a patient who initially presents with a Functional Communication Measure of 3 in a skilled nursing facility, what level has the patient attained when treatment is concluded?
- How many sessions did it take to achieve that goal?
- How many treatment units were rendered to reach that goal?
- Is there a difference in the amount of progress made by patients who enter at that level in an outpatient setting as compared to a rehabilitation hospital? A long-term care facility?

As the NOMS becomes even more sophisticated, it will be able to track patients through the continuum of care rather than just segments of care. At that point, extremely valuable information will be available to answer these questions:

- At what period within the continuum of care (acute care to rehabilitation facility to home care) did the patient demonstrate the most progress according to a functional measure?
- If patients are on tube feeding in acute care, at what stage in the continuum of care do they reach a level (4 or 5) at which they no longer need tube feeding?
- At what point in the continuum of care are patients eating a nearly normal diet (level 6)?
- What percentage of patients return to eating a nearly normal diet?
- How do we answer these questions related to different patients' diagnoses?

In order to answer these very specific questions, ASHA will need a great deal of data in the database.

Short-Term Goals

Short-term goals are those that one expects to reach within a specified period of time (such as one month, two weeks). Too often, these goals are written in terms that are not functional, and they are not meaningful to others. Examples of functional and nonfunctional short-term goals are presented in Table 4–2.

After setting long- and short-term goals, the clinician must decide whether the patient can safely eat anything by mouth. If the patient cannot, the clinician will need to select only indirect treatment methods. Logemann (1998b) indicates that this means the patient is at great risk for aspiration and that no compensatory techniques, postural changes, or diet changes have been found that will allow the patient to swallow anything safely. If they

Table 4–2 Functional and Nonfunctional Short-Term Goals

Goal Written in Nonfunctional Terms	*Goal Written in Functional Terms*
1. Patient will improve strength of lip closure.	1. Patient will keep food and liquid in the mouth while eating without losing it out the front of the mouth.
2. Patient will increase strength and coordination of tongue muscles.	2a. Patient will be able to put food into a cohesive bolus to reduce the risk of the food falling over the back of the tongue. OR 2b. Patient will be able to move the cohesive bolus of food to the back of the mouth and through the hypopharynx to reduce the risk of parts of the bolus falling into the airway. OR 2c. Patient will be able to keep bolus in the mouth until ready to swallow, so that the airway will be better protected.
3. Patient will increase speed of initiation of swallow.	3. Patient will decrease the delay in initiation of pharyngeal swallow to decrease the risk of liquid or food falling into the airway during a delay.
4. Patient will increase laryngeal closure.	4. Patient will reduce the risk of food entering the airway by achieving better closure of the airway at the larynx.
5. Patient will increase laryngeal elevation.	5. Patient will reduce the risk of food entering the airway by increasing laryngeal elevation.

cannot swallow anything safely, you will need to select indirect treatment methods. If the patient can eat by mouth, it is more desirable to do direct therapy (involving presentation of food and/or liquid). Swallowing is the best practice for swallowing. Swallowing something is also a much more functional activity than practicing swallowing with saliva only.

Treatment Objectives

Treatment objectives are the small, measurable steps to achieve short-term goals. Treatment objectives are not typically written in functional terms, because they are based on deficits. One identifies the problem/deficit and writes a treatment objective to improve that deficit. Examples of treatment objectives for short-term goals listed are presented in Exhibit 4–7.

The activities used to achieve treatment objectives can be divided into three basic categories:

1. *Compensatory.* These strategies can include changes in posture and increasing sensory input before or during the swallow. Food placement and presentation are designed to compensate for the patient's deficits. These strategies are used during meals or therapeutic feeding.
2. *Facilitation techniques.* These techniques are designed to actually improve function and can be considered therapeutic exercises. For example, breath hold (or Valsalva maneuver) is designed to increase strength of vocal cord closure. Some facilitation techniques are also used as compensatory techniques. For example, the Mendelsohn maneuver facilitates elevation of the larynx. It can also be used as a compensation during swallowing to maintain laryngeal elevation to reduce residue in the pyriform sinuses.
3. *Diet.* A final category of strategies is change in diet. This includes changing the texture of foods and thickness of liquids. It can also involve presenting different tastes and temperatures.

Short-term goals and treatment objectives should be based on the patient's physiology, not just the symptoms observed. For example, the symptom of residue in valleculae might be observed in two patients for very different reasons. One patient might have residue because of decreased base of tongue and posterior pharyngeal wall pressure. The other

Exhibit 4–7 Sample Short-Term Goals and Treatment Objectives

Short-Term Goal	*Examples of Treatment Objectives*
1. Patient will keep food and liquid in the mouth without losing any out the front.	• Patient will achieve lip closure against resistance provided by clinician placing fingers on upper and lower lip on 8 of 10 trials (F). • Patient will avoid foods in liquid base without cues (D).
2a. Patient will be able to put food into a cohesive bolus to keep food from falling over the back of the tongue into the airway.	• Patient will place bolus of food on stronger side with cues on 8 of 10 trials (C). • Patient will push right/left lateral border of tongue against tongue blade on 7 of 10 trials (F).
2b. Patient will be able to move the cohesive bolus of food to the back of the mouth and through the hypopharnyx to reduce the risk of parts of the bolus falling into the airway.	• Patient will move tip of tongue from alveolar ridge to border of soft palate on 8 of 10 trials (F). • Patient will eat only foods that form cohesive bolus (D).
2c. Patient will be able to keep bolus in the mouth until ready to swallow to reduce chance of food falling into the airway.	• Patient will use chin-down posture for thin consistencies with cues on 10 of 10 trials (C). • Patient will produce forceful K sound at end of words on 9 of 10 trials (F).
3. Patient will decrease delay in initiation of pharnygeal swallow to reduce risk of food or liquid falling into the airway during the delay.	• Patient will decrease length of time from command to swallow to onset of swallow from 5 seconds to 2 seconds following thermal-tactile stimulation (F, C).
4. Patient will reduce the risk of food falling into the airway by improving closure of the larynx.	• Patient will use head rotation to left with cues on 10 of 10 trials (C).

continues

Exhibit 4–7 continued

	• Patient will demonstrate Valsalva maneuver (breath hold) on 8 of 10 trials (F).
5. Patient will decrease risk of food falling into the airway by increasing laryngeal elevation.	• Patient will control bolus size to teaspoon amounts with cues on 10 of 10 trials (C). • Patient will demonstrate Mendelsohn maneuver on 5 of 10 trials (F, C).
Key: Objectives are identified as facilitation (F), compensation (C), or diet (D).	

patient might have vallecular residue because of limited laryngeal elevation. Different goals and treatment objectives would be selected for these patients, even though they have the same symptom.

DETERMINING READINESS FOR DISCHARGE

With the constraints placed on services by limitations in reimbursement, it is more important than ever to begin planning for discharge from the initial contact with the patient. Selecting a long-term goal is basically giving a prognosis for that patient. Can this patient return to eating by mouth? If so, will all nutrition and hydration needs be met by mouth or will supplemental tube feeding always be needed? Is this patient going to be able to eat a normal diet? Or is the patient clearly not a candidate to take any more than a few bites or sips here and there? Each of these patients has a very different prognosis.

Reimbursement constraints may also mean setting long-term goals to help the patient achieve a functional outcome rather than an optimal outcome. The following example may help explain the difference between functional and optimal:

> The patient is seen in an acute rehabilitation setting after a stroke. He is admitted with a nasogastric tube still in place but has been deemed safe to swallow pudding-thick liquids in teaspoon amounts with several compensatory techniques and maximum cues to use

these techniques. After three weeks of treatment, he is reassessed via videofluoroscopy and found to be safe on a mechanical soft diet as long as all fruits and vegetables are drained of excess liquid and have a cohesive consistency. He can take syrup-thick liquids in uncontrolled amounts, or thin liquids in teaspoon amounts if he uses a chin-down technique and receives moderate cues to do so.

Is the patient achieving a functional outcome yet? He is certainly not achieving an optimal outcome. If the goal is for this patient to be home alone, with someone else to come in and prepare meals, then he might be safe to eat by himself as long as the foods and liquids were prepared appropriately. He would probably need to be presented with syrup-thick liquids only, because no one would be there to provide the necessary cuing to use his compensatory techniques. However, if the goal for this patient is to return to work, and part of his job is holding daily sales meetings over lunch, then this level may not be functional for the patient.

The speech-language pathologist should begin counseling the patient and family from the onset of treatment about realistic expectations. It is important to help them understand the payment limitations as well and, when appropriate, to offer to help them seek other services or funding sources when payment reimbursement is discontinued. It is also possible to establish a treatment plan the family can follow when the patient must be discharged due to financial constraints.

ETHICAL ISSUES

Some of these issues about functional and realistic outcomes may lead to an ethical dilemma. The "Code of Ethics" of the American Speech-Language-Hearing Association (ASHA, 1994) provides some guidance. According to the code, "Individuals shall honor their responsibility to hold paramount the welfare of persons they serve professionally" (p. 1). Two specific rules of ethics may provide some guidance when dealing with ethical dilemmas.

- *Rule D:* Individuals shall fully inform the persons they serve of the nature and possible effects of services rendered and products dispensed.

- *Rule F:* Individuals shall not guarantee the results of any treatment or procedure, directly or by implication; however, they may make a reasonable statement of prognosis (p. 1).

Below are several examples of cases involving functional outcomes that may require the speech-language pathologist to call upon the "Code of Ethics" for guidance.

- The speech-language pathologist has screened the patient at bedside; she shows several clinical signs of aspiration, and she has advanced dementia. The speech-language pathologist recommends an instrumental assessment to determine if there is anything the patient can eat safely; the physician refuses to write the order, stating that the patient is not expected to improve, so why bother with an expensive evaluation? He writes an order instead for the speech-language pathologist to feed whatever she thinks is the safest diet. The speech-language pathologist suspects that the patient cannot eat anything safely and, even if she could, the clinician does not think she can maintain nutrition and hydration with the small amount she will take. Should the speech-language pathologist feed the patient?
- The patient is in the advanced stages of dementia when the speech-language pathologist performs a modified barium swallow (MBS) study. The test reveals the patient is aspirating everything, and no compensatory strategies can eliminate the aspiration. The patient has an advance directive indicating that he does not want a feeding tube of any kind. What does the practitioner tell the family members who care for this patient at home?
- The patient has had a brainstem CVA and presents with a severely delayed swallow and is aspirating. The speech-language pathologist explains that she has a good prognosis for returning to some food by mouth safely. She is refusing treatment and tube feeding. Does the practitioner try to change her mind or honor her wishes?

IMPROVING MEDICAL OUTCOMES

The ultimate functional outcome of dysphagia management is to affect the patient's overall health status. The most obvious impact of dysphagia management on the patient's medical condition is the prevention of aspiration pneumonia. The cost to treat an aspiration pneumonia has been estimated at $10,000 to $15,000 depending on the area of the country (Logemann, 1998a). Evaluation and treatment of dysphagia, which can prevent aspiration pneumonia, is both medically effective and cost beneficial.

Appropriate and effective assessment and treatment of swallowing disorders have been shown to improve the health, safety, and quality of life for patients with dysphagia. For example, Kasprisin, Clumeck, and Nino-Murcia (1989) found that only 15% of adult patients with dysphagia and a history of aspiration pneumonia experienced a recurrence in the one-year period following rehabilitative management of their swallowing problems, while aspiration pneumonia occurred in 75% of untreated patients in the one-year period following diagnosis.

Some linkages between dysphagia management and overall health of the patient are not as obvious. However, patients with dysphagia may experience malnutrition. Malnutrition increases healing time of wounds and increases hospital length of stay.

CONCLUSION

Dysphagia management provides the speech-language pathologist the opportunity to make a significant difference in the quality of a patient's life. It can result in rapid and significant change in the patient's ability to swallow safely, changing his or her ability to participate in one of the most functional activities of our daily lives—eating. Consider this patient's description of the impact of dysphagia intervention: "When I had my G-tube, I didn't even want to sit at the table with the rest of the family while they were eating. I felt like an outcast. I couldn't go out to restaurants with friends and just eat pudding while they enjoyed a full meal. Now that I am eating again, I feel like I have my life back."

Who can imagine a more functional outcome than that!

Discussion Questions

1. Why should speech-language pathologists focus on reporting functional outcomes?
2. How can detailed information be obtained about a person's swallowing disorder?

3. What are possible consequences of treating a patient with pharyngeal dysphagia without an instrumental assessment?
4. How can rating scales of swallowing function be used with instrumental assessments?
5. What is the difference between a short-term goal and a treatment objective?

REFERENCES

American Speech-Language-Hearing Association. (1994). Code of ethics. *Asha, 36* (Suppl. 13), 1–2.

American Speech-Language-Hearing Association. (1998). *National outcomes measurement system: Functional communication measures*. Rockville, MD: Author.

Garon, B.R., Engle, M., & Ormiston, C. (1996). Silent aspiration: Results of 1000 videofluoroscopic swallowing evaluations. *Journal of Neurologic Rehabilitation, 10*, 121–126.

Gordon, C., Hewer, R., & Weda, D. (1987). Dysphagia and acute stroke. *British Medical Journal, 195*, 411–414.

Horner, J., Riski, J.E., Ovelmen-Levitt, J., & Nashold, B.S. (1992). Swallowing in torticollis before and after rhizotomy. *Dysphagia, 7* (3), 117–125.

Kasprisin, A., Clumeck, H., & Nino-Murcia, M. (1989). The efficacy of rehabilitative management of dysphagia. *Dysphagia 4,* 48–52.

Langmore, S.E. (1998). Instrumental assessment of dysphagia: Fluoroscopy or FEES®? Paper presented at the 1998 Kentucky Conference of Communication Disorders, Louisville, KY.

Leder, S. (1996). Comments on Thompson-Henry and Braddock: The modified Evan's blue dye procedure for us to detect aspiration in the tracheotomized patient: Five case reports. *Dysphagia, 11*, 80–81.

Logemann, J. (1998a). *Dysphagia Audio Digest, 5* (1). Gaylord, MI: Northern Speech Services.

Logemann, J. (1998b). *Evaluation and treatment of swallowing disorders* (2nd ed.). Austin, TX: ProEd.

Loughlin, G. (1989). Respiratory consequences of dysfunctional swallowing and aspiration. *Dysphagia, 3*, 126–130.

Lugger, K. (1994). Dysphagia in the elderly stroke patient. *Journal of Neuroscience Nursing, 26* (*2*), 78–84.

Murray, J., Langmore, S., Ginsberg, S., & Dostie, A. (1996). The significance of accumulated oropharyngeal secretions and swallowing frequency in predicting aspiration. *Dysphagia, 11*, 99–103.

Rosenbek, J., Robbins, J., Roecker, E., Coyle, J., & Wood, J. (1996). A penetration-aspiration scale, *Dysphagia, 11*, 93–98

Splaingard, M., Hutchins, B., Sulton, L., & Chaudhuri, G. (1988, August). Aspiration in rehabilitation patients: Videofluoroscopy versus bedside clinical assessment. *Archives of Physical Medicine and Rehabilitation*, *69*, 637–640.

Spray, S., Zuidema, G., Cameron, J. (1976). Aspiration pneumonia: Incidents of aspiration with endotracheal tubes. *American Journal of Surgery, 131*, 701–703.

Steefel, J. (1981). *Dysphagia rehabilitation for neurologically impaired adults*. Springfield, IL: Charles C. Thomas.

Swigert, N. (1996). *The source for dysphagia*. East Moline, IL: LinguiSystems,

Terry, B., & Fuller, S. (1989). Pulmonary consequences of aspiration. *Dysphagia, 3*, 179–183.

Thompson-Henry, S., & Braddock, B. (1995). The modified Evans blue dye procedure fails to detect aspiration in the tracheotomized patient: Five case reports. *Dysphagia, 10*, 172–174.

Tippett, D.C., & Siebens, A.A. (1996). Reconsidering the value of the modified Evans blue dye test: A comment on Thomson-Henry and Braddock. *Dysphagia, 11*, 78–79.

Uniform Data System for Medical Rehabilitation. (1995). *Guide for the use of the uniform data system for medical rehabilitation (Adult FIM), version 4.0*. Buffalo, NY: State University of New York at Buffalo.

Young, E.C., & Durant-Jones, L. (1997). Gradual onset of dysphagia: A study of patients with oculopharyngeal muscular dystrophy. *Dysphagia, 12*, 196–201.

Zenner, P.M., Losinski, D.S., & Mills, R.H. (1995). Using cervical auscultation in the clinical dysphagia examination in long-term care. *Dysphagia, 10* (*1*), 27–31.

SUGGESTED READINGS

Logemann, J. (1998). *Evaluation and treatment of swallowing disorders*. Austin, TX: Pro-Ed.

Sonies, B. (1997). *Dysphagia: A continuum of care*. Gaithersburg, MD: Aspen Publishers, Inc.

Swigert, N. (1996). *The source for dysphagia*. East Moline, IL: LinguiSystems.

Swigert, N. (1998). *The source for pediatric dysphagia*. East Moline, IL: LinguiSystems.

CHAPTER 5

An Everyday Approach to Long-Term Rehabilitation after Traumatic Brain Injury

Mark Ylvisaker, James Feeney, and Timothy J. Feeney

Objectives

- Describe the consequences of frontolimbic injury.
- Describe alternative approaches to impairment, disability, and handicap in cognitive rehabilitation.
- Provide a rationale for contextualized, collaborative, hypothesis-testing assessment as a basis for intervention.
- Illustrate contextualized, routine-based cognitive and behavioral intervention for people with traumatic brain injury.

INTRODUCTION

The goal of this chapter is to describe, illustrate, and promote an approach to rehabilitation that has evolved over the course of our work with more than 1,000 children, adolescents, and adults with chronic impairment after traumatic brain injury (TBI). After sketching common ability profiles of people with TBI, we offer a framework for providing rehabilitation services and supports to people with chronic impairment in domains of functioning in which cognition, communication, behavior, and executive functions overlap. We offer a neuropsychological rationale for this approach to intervention and then connect this neuropsychological orientation to Vygotsky's theory of cognitive development. Much of the chapter is devoted to two case illustrations designed to show concretely how rehabilitative intervention can be delivered within a contextualized, everyday, routine-based approach.

FUNCTIONAL IMPAIRMENT AFTER TRAUMATIC BRAIN INJURY

TBI is an unusual and in some ways unhelpful disability category. Virtually any outcome is possible after TBI, depending on a variety of factors, including the following:

- the person's age at the time of injury
- the person's preinjury ability profile, personality, accomplishments, adjustment, and support systems
- the nature, location, and severity of the brain injury
- other injuries
- emergency medical management
- early medical and rehabilitative care
- postinjury support systems, including quality of long-term rehabilitative, educational, and vocational supports
- postinjury support systems, including resiliency and competence of family members, friends, coworkers, and others
- the individual's evolving emotional and psychosocial adjustment

Despite this noteworthy diversity, there are interesting central tendencies within the population, based on (1) the preinjury vulnerabilities in the group of people most at risk for TBI (often young, risk-taking males) and (2) the relative vulnerability of specific parts of the brain in closed head injury, which is the most common cause of TBI. It has long been known that frontolimbic structures (especially prefrontal lobe and subcortical medial temporal lobe limbic structures, including the hippocampus) are most vulnerable in closed-head injury, regardless of site of impact on the skull, if acceleration/deceleration forces are created within the skull and if there is secondary anoxic injury (Adams, Graham, Scott, Parker, & Doyle, 1980; Levin, Goldstein, Williams, & Eisenberg, 1991; Mendelsohn et al., 1992). Elsewhere we have described in detail the impairment associated with damage to these parts of the brain (Ylvisaker & Feeney, 1998a). Exhibit 5–1 outlines frequently observed impairments associated with frontolimbic damage, grouped under four headings: executive system impairment, communication impairment, cognitive impairment, and behavioral impairment. Several publications in the research literature summarize language outcome in children and adults with TBI (Biddle, McCabe,

Exhibit 5–1 Vulnerable Frontolimbic Structures and Frequently Associated Impairments

FRONTOLIMBIC INJURY AND EXECUTIVE SYSTEM IMPAIRMENT

- reduced awareness of personal strengths and weaknesses
- difficulty setting realistic goals
- difficulty planning and organizing behavior to achieve the goals
- impaired ability to initiate action needed to achieve the goals
- difficulty inhibiting behavior incompatible with achieving the goals
- difficulty self-monitoring and self-evaluating
- difficulty thinking strategically and solving real-world problems in a flexible and efficient manner
- general inflexibility and concreteness in thinking and acting

FRONTOLIMBIC INJURY AND COMMUNICATION IMPAIRMENT

- disorganized, poorly controlled discourse or paucity of discourse (spoken and written)
- inefficient comprehension of language related to increasing amounts of information to be processed (spoken or written) and to rate of speech
- word retrieval problems
- difficulty understanding and expressing abstract and indirect language
- difficulty interpreting speaker's intent in social contexts
- awkward or inappropriate communication in stressful social contexts
- impaired verbal learning

FRONTOLIMBIC INJURY AND COGNITIVE IMPAIRMENT

- reduced internal control over all cognitive functions (e.g., attentional, perceptual, memory, organizational, and reasoning processes)
- impaired working memory
- impaired declarative and explicit memory (encoding and retrieval)
- disorganized behavior related to impaired organizing schemes (managerial knowledge frames, such as scripts, themes, schemas, mental models)
- impaired reasoning
- concrete thinking
- difficulty generalizing

FRONTOLIMBIC INJURY AND BEHAVIORAL IMPAIRMENT

- disinhibited, socially inappropriate, and possibly aggressive behavior
- impaired initiation or paucity of behavior
- inefficient learning from consequences
- perseverative behavior
- impaired social perception and interpretation

& Bliss, 1996; Chapman, 1997; Chapman et al., 1995, 1997; Dennis, 1991, 1992; Dennis & Barnes, 1990; Dennis, Barnes, Donnelly, Wilkinson, & Humphreys, 1996; Dennis & Lovett, 1990; Groher, 1990; Hagen, 1981; Hartley, 1995; Liles, Coelho, Duffy, & Zalagens, 1989; McDonald, 1992a, 1992b, 1993; Mentis & Prutting, 1991; Sarno, Buonaguro, & Levita, 1986; Turkstra & Holland, 1998; Ylvisaker, 1992, 1993).

In examining lists like those presented in Exhibit 5–1, it is critical to recognize that, in most cases, impairments listed under one heading are simply alternative labels for or manifestations of impairments listed under other headings. For example, disinhibition (executive system impairment) often manifests itself as a social communication or pragmatic impairment from a communication perspective, as aggressive or otherwise socially inappropriate behavior from a behavioral perspective, and as immature reasoning or superficial encoding of information from a cognitive perspective. Damage to frontal lobe organizational centers may appear as a planning deficit (executive functions), impaired organizational thinking and disorganized encoding and retrieval of information (cognition), weak comprehension and expression of extended discourse (communication), and socially awkward behavior in the absence of well-rehearsed routines (behavior). Frank recognition of the seamless garment that is executive system-communication-cognitive-behavioral impairment after TBI leads directly and ineluctably to an enthusiastic endorsement of fiercely collaborative intervention. It makes no sense for professionals from varied disciplines to approach essentially the same underlying issues from separate and potentially fragmenting perspectives.

A FUNCTIONAL, EVERYDAY APPROACH TO INTERVENTION AND SUPPORT

In referring to a favored approach to intervention as *functional*, one flirts with an unfortunate disingenuity. Calling one approach functional suggests that alternative approaches are *nonfunctional*. Yet an exhaustive search is unlikely to uncover a single helping professional who would willingly identify his or her approach to intervention as nonfunctional. To be a helping professional is to be a person who attempts to help others who are sick or who have a disability to function better. All responsible clinicians deliver what they consider functional intervention.

The ultimate clinical question, then, is this: What approach or approaches to intervention for a given individual or disability group help that person or those people to function most successfully in relation to their goals and life context? This is a very difficult question to answer in the case of people with a complex disability like that commonly associated with severe TBI. However, some answers to the question are clearly wrong. For example, it will not do to answer the question in a superficial manner. (For example, "Approach *X* is most functional because it is delivered in the person's home or [in the case of children] because the activities are fun for the child.") Nor is it acceptable to answer the question in an apparently more scientific manner: "Approach *X* is most functional because it is the only approach supported by controlled clinical trials with this population." Nor is it acceptable to answer the question in a trendy, consumer-oriented manner: "I do exactly what my clients (patients, students) direct me to do; that's functional."

Decisions about how most effectively to help individuals with chronic disability necessitate thoughtful consideration of many factors. In domains of impairment in which the need for clinical services is undeniable, but published experimental guidance is incomplete, responsible clinicians must make decisions about intervention for specific individuals with disability based on informed consideration of the following factors:

- Is the proposed intervention supported by intervention outcome studies with subjects from the same diagnostic category and who possess the same impairments and needs as the client?
- Is the proposed intervention supported by intervention outcome studies with related populations (such as learning disabilities, developmental disabilities, attention deficit/hyperactivity disorder)?
- Is the proposed intervention supported by trial intervention with the client?
- Is the proposed intervention supported by extensive clinical experience with the client's population?
- Is the proposed intervention supported by theory, including neuropsychological, cognitive, behavioral, pedagogical, and other theories?
- Is the proposed intervention supported by negotiation with the client and relevant stakeholders in the client's life?

- Is the proposed intervention consistent with known constraints, including expertise of service providers, availability of support personnel, time to complete the intervention, and adequate resources?
- Can the proposed intervention be judged to be preferable to known alternatives—in relation to predicted functional outcome for the client—based on the previous considerations?
- Is the proposed intervention humane, morally justifiable, and consistent with the scope of practice and relevant licensing laws governing the provider of services?

In our experience with several hundred children, adolescents, and adults with chronic disability after TBI—disability in the territory in which communication, cognition, executive functions, and behavior overlap, interact, and become essentially indistinguishable—the approach outlined and illustrated in this chapter is typically most functional.

Theoretical Foundations

Damasio (1994) has clearly identified the many obstacles to success in life encountered by people with significant frontolimbic injury. Figure 5–1 illustrates his important summary of neuropsychological findings in the form of a dilemma. People succeed in social, educational, and vocational pursuits because (1) they are capable of making thoughtful and effective decisions about how to act, (2) their behavior has been positively shaped by their history of successes and failures (rewards and punishments)—or, in most cases, (3) they combine thoughtful decision making and effective habits shaped by their reinforcement history. Unfortunately, severe frontolimbic injury often compromises both routes to successful action.

As outlined in Figure 5–1, frontal lobe injury often results in the following problems: some degree of dissociation between thinking and acting; concrete thinking and impaired reasoning; weak organizing and planning; impulsiveness; difficulty transferring; impaired working memory; possibly reduced initiation; and weak deliberate, strategic learning. Thus, successful action by means of high reason is threatened, which creates the first horn of the dilemma. Unfortunately, learning from consequences is also impaired in many people with frontal lobe injury. According to Damasio, stored memories (however conscious or unconscious) are capable of guiding future decision making only if those memories combine two distinct components: (1) the intellectual component (such as remembering that arriving late at work resulted in a reprimand and loss of a

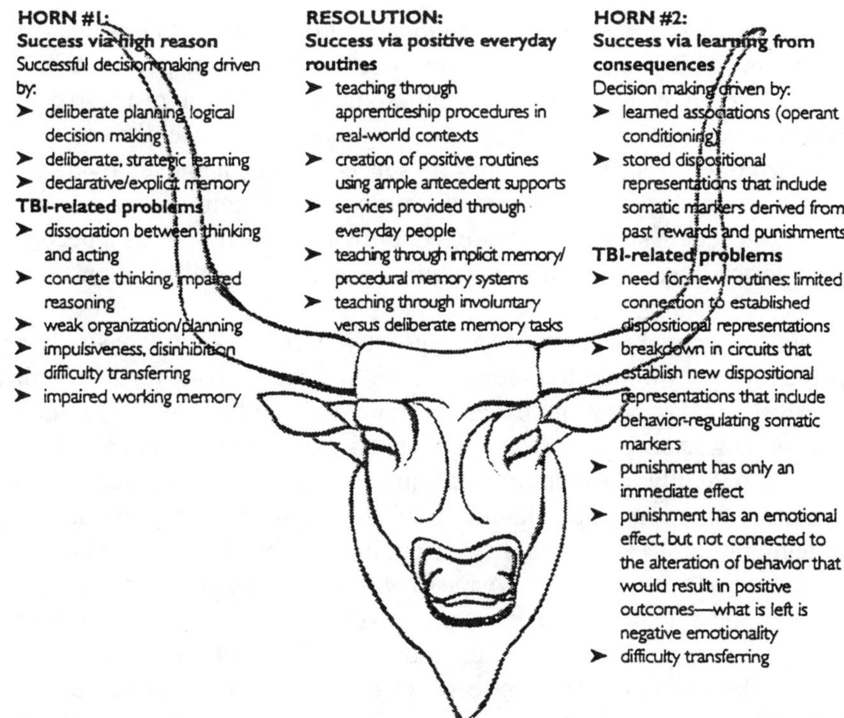

Figure 5–1 A TBI dilemma and its proposed resolution. *Source:* Reprinted with permission from M. Ylvisaker and T. Feeney, *Collaborative Brain Injury Intervention: Positive Everyday Routines*, © 1998, Singular Publishing Group.

promised raise) and (2) the "somatic marker" or feeling state that is capable of driving future behavior (the gut-level sense, "That was not a good thing!"). Damasio's neuropsychological investigations suggest that ventromedial prefrontal cortex is critical to the circuitry that creates stored representations that include behavior-guiding somatic markers. Ventral prefrontal cortex may be the most vulnerable part of the brain in closed head injury. Others argue that it is impulsiveness associated with orbitofrontal injuries that results in inefficiency in learning from consequences (Rolls, Hornack, Wade, & McGrath, 1994). Still others have found impaired working memory to be associated with weak learning from consequences (Alderman, 1996). Whatever the best explanation, this is the second horn of the dilemma.

The question facing rehabilitation specialists is, "How are we to help people whose thought processes are weak and poorly connected to their practical decisions and who are also inefficient at learning from the consequences of their actions?" An *unacceptable* answer to this question, but one implicitly embraced by many specialists and nonspecialists alike, is that people who fit this description must live in a restrictive and protected environment in which other people play the role of their "prosthetic frontal lobes." On the contrary, success can be achieved by helping people establish positive, everyday routines of thought and action, with ample antecedent supports that are withdrawn systematically as it becomes possible to do so. This chapter is an elaboration and illustration of this thesis.

Ylvisaker and Feeney (1998a) presented Vygotsky's increasingly respected theory of cognitive development as a framework for facilitating improvement in cognition, executive functions, and related communication and behavioral competencies. Vygotsky viewed most cognitive processes (e.g., deliberate memory, reasoning, organizing) and executive self-regulatory functions (e.g., planning, deliberate inhibition, self-monitoring, strategic thinking) as having their origin in the everyday social-communication routines that children engage in with their parents, other adults, and more competent children. That is, processes such as organizing, planning, remembering, problem solving, and strategic thinking first exist as interpsychological or social processes—as interaction between a child or other apprentice in thinking and a more mature person. Gradually, the processes are internalized and ultimately come to exist as internal cognitive and executive system processes (Vygotsky, 1978, 1981).

Clearly there is a universe of detail and complexity within this view that is beyond the scope of this chapter. However, Exhibit 5–2 outlines key differences between the structure of teaching tasks dictated by the traditional training model of instruction (with which most helping professionals are very familiar) and the structure of teaching tasks dictated by a Vygotskyan apprenticeship model. The case illustrations presented later in this chapter are designed to further illuminate this approach to rehabilitation.

Sources of Support for an Everyday, Routine-Based Approach to Rehabilitation

During the initial period of intensive program development in TBI rehabilitation, extending from the mid-1970s through the 1980s, rehabilitation specialists expressed considerable enthusiasm for an approach to

Exhibit 5–2 Features of Teaching Tasks: Traditional Training Model Versus Vygotskyan Apprenticeship Model

TRADITIONAL TRAINING MODEL

Context

- Training takes place outside of a natural setting.
- Performance of the learner is demanded by the trainer.
- Performance is solo, not social.
- Tasks and components of tasks are hierarchically organized.

Task Structure

- The trainer requests performance of a specific task.
- The trainer may model performance.
- The learner performs.
- If the performance is adequate, the learner is reinforced.
- If the performance is inadequate, the trainer does one of the following:
  –requests a hierarchically easier task
  –reduces the difficulty of the task
  –provides needed cues, prompts, shaping procedures
- When performance is adequate, repeated practice is required to habituate the learned behavior.
- Systematic transfer procedures are then applied.

VYGOTSKYAN APPRENTICESHIP MODEL

Context

- Learning (ideally) takes place in a natural setting for the behavior or skill that is to be learned.
- Learning takes place within the context of projects designed to achieve a meaningful goal.
- Performance is not demanded from the learner; rather the task is completed collaboratively.
- Completion of the task is social, not solo.
- The learner is not expected to fail; the collaborator is available to contribute whatever the learner cannot contribute to successful completion of the task.
- Tasks are not necessarily organized hierarchically; the learner can learn aspects of difficult tasks by participating with a collaborator.

continues

Exhibit 5–2 continued

Task Structure

- The teacher (facilitator, collaborator) introduces a task and engages the learner in guided observation (not necessarily task specific).
- The teacher engages the learner in collaborative, functional, goal-oriented, project-oriented work.
- The learner contributes what he or she can contribute.
- The teacher coaches (including suggestions, modeling, brainstorming, cues, feedback, and encouragement) and continues to collaborate as the learner accomplishes more components of the task.
- As the learner improves, supports are systematically withdrawn or the task is made more difficult or both.
- The teacher continues to provide ongoing incidental coaching.
- Transfer is guaranteed because it is part of the contextualized teaching process from the beginning.

Source: Reprinted with permission from M. Ylvisaker and T. Feeney, *Collaborative Brain Injury Intervention: Positive Everyday Routines*, © 1998, Singular Publishing Group.

rehabilitation quite different from that described in this chapter. Popular interventions targeted the underlying cognitive, behavioral, and communication impairment; were delivered by specialists working in relative isolation; and were delivered in clinical settings using training tasks largely unrelated to the individual's real-world tasks and stressors. Thus, for example, cognitive rehabilitation came to be understood by many practitioners as an enterprise based on precise neuropsychological delineation of the individual's underlying impairments, followed by an intensive program of hierarchically organized exercises designed to remediate those impairments (e.g., Sohlberg & Mateer, 1989). In the early stages of clinical research, success was measured by improvement on training tasks or neuropsychological tests. Using this measure of success, cognitive retraining exercises seemed to have an important treatment effect (e.g., Ruff et al., 1989). However, in some areas (such as memory retraining), that effect has been found to be clinically insignificant (Schacter & Glisky, 1986); in others, important questions have been raised about reduction of impairment and transfer from training tasks to real-world application (e.g., Ponsford, 1990).

Our enthusiasm about an everyday, routine-based approach to rehabilitation is based on (1) extensive clinical experience with a large number of individuals with TBI, (2) a limited amount of experimental research with this population (e.g., Feeney & Ylvisaker, 1995; Finset & Andresen, 1990; von Cramon & Mathes-von Cramon, 1994; Ylvisaker & Feeney, 1998a), (3) the neuropsychological and developmental theories described in the last section, (4) the extensive literature dealing with transfer of training in both behavioral and cognitive psychology, (5) an impressive body of intervention research in related fields of intervention, and (6) the managed care mandate to generate quality outcomes with dramatically shrinking resources.

With respect to transfer of training, many investigators in behavioral and cognitive psychology have amassed evidence that supports the following heuristic principle: *Behaviors or skills acquired in a laboratory or training context are unlikely to transfer to functional application contexts and be maintained over time without heroic efforts to facilitate that transfer and maintenance* (Horner, Dunlap, & Koegel, 1988; Martin & Pear, 1996; Morris, 1992; Singley & Anderson, 1989). Recognition of the impact of this principle has led to the development and validation of increasingly contextualized interventions in many clinical fields, including vocational rehabilitation (e.g., Wehman et al., 1993, 1995), special education (e.g., Giangreco, Cloninger, & Iverson, 1993), strategy intervention for students with and without specific disability (e.g., Pressley, 1995), behavioral intervention (e.g., Carr, Levin, McConnachie, Carlson, Kemp, & Smith, 1994; Carr, Reeve, & Magito-McLaughlin, 1997; Kennedy, 1994; Koegel, Koegel, & Dunlap, 1997; Reichle & Wacker, 1993), and language and social skills intervention (e.g., Fey, 1986; Koegel & Koegel, 1995; MacDonald, 1989; Walker et al., 1994; Wiener & Harris, 1998).

Impairment, Disability, and Handicap in Brain Injury Rehabilitation

In an attempt to systematize thinking and talking about disability and rehabilitation, the World Health Organization (WHO, 1980) proposed definitions of impairment, disability, and handicap. Within this classification system, *impairment* refers to the underlying damage to psychological, physiological, or anatomic structures or functions (such as aphasia associated with perisylvian left hemisphere stroke); *disability* refers to an associated reduction in the ability to perform functional activities in a normal manner (such as difficulty finding words in conversation); and *handicap* refers to the social, educational, vocational, or other role disadvantage associated with the disability (such as failure in school or loss of a job due to the communication impairment).

As indicated in Exhibit 5–3, traditional rehabilitation—including physical, cognitive, communication, and psychosocial rehabilitation—focuses initially on reducing the individual's underlying impairment, often with decontextualized exercises targeting underlying and purportedly general neuropsychological processes. If impairment-oriented intervention is successful, then disability and associated handicap are thereby eliminated. For obvious reasons, this is the ideal in rehabilitation. However, after severe TBI, some degree of impairment and associated disability almost always persists, even with a lengthy and intensive program of impairment-oriented restorative exercises. Therefore, attempts to reduce the associated disability with compensatory procedures may be introduced as a second-best treatment option. If this effort is insufficiently successful, then the focus shifts to handicap-oriented interventions, putting supports in place for the individual and modifying the expectations of key people in the environment. This final effort is often thought to represent failure and is therefore a last resort. The traditional progression has been shown to be important in treating certain types of sensory and motor impairment after brain injury. Indeed, in some cases, it is necessary to *prevent* people from using compensations (disability-oriented intervention) in the interest of attacking the underlying impairment.

In contrast to this traditional progression, the approach we describe is one in which social, academic, and/or vocational handicap is attacked first, with task modifications and external supports designed to enable the person to be successful. With extensive contextualized practice in the use of compensatory procedures and aids, and systematic reduction in external support, the individual may then experience a reduction in disability. That is, using special procedures, devices, or effort, the person with ongoing impairment becomes able to complete functional tasks that were previously impossible or required considerable support from others. Finally, in some cases, ongoing contextualized practice with the compensations results in their internalization, producing a reduction in underlying impairment as the individual performs more effectively without needing to deliberately use compensatory procedures or other special efforts.

The last point—ultimate reduction of impairment—is worth underscoring. Many people erroneously characterize a functional approach to rehabilitation as one that focuses on handicap and disability *as opposed to*

Exhibit 5–3 Two Perspectives on the Relations Between Impairment-Oriented, Disability-Oriented, and Handicap-Oriented Interventions

TRADITIONAL REHABILITATION

Step 1: Attempt to eliminate the individual's underlying impairment with impairment-oriented treatment tasks.

Step 2: Attempt to reduce functional disability with compensatory procedures if impairment-oriented treatment is insufficiently successful.

Step 3: Attempt to reduce social, vocational, and/or educational handicap if impairment- and disability-oriented interventions are insufficiently successful.

AN ALTERNATIVE PERSPECTIVE

Step 1: Reduce handicap by modifying everyday routines, including the support provided by everyday people in the environment.

Step 2: Potentially decrease disability by including functional compensatory procedures in the individual's everyday routines and ensuring intensive contextualized practice in the use of those compensatory procedures.

Step 3: Potentially reduce the impairment by ensuring that the individual practices compensatory procedures—in increasingly varied contexts—to the point at which they are internalized and become components of his or her automatic cognitive or self-regulatory mechanism.

impairment. We propose, in contrast, that the focus on handicap and disability is part of a long-term process that often—though not always—results in reduction of impairment *in addition to and as a result of* reduction in handicap and disability. Both case illustrations presented later in this chapter progress in this way from reduction of handicap to reduction of disability to reduction of impairment. For example, in the first case a male adult initially required intensive external supports and reminders (such as self-talk routines modeled by staff) to avoid disinhibited and aggressive social behavior; with this support in place, his handicap was reduced. Gradually, staff members were able to reduce the frequency of their reminders as the client assumed responsibility for deliberate self-reminders. Finally, self-reminders became so habitual that they were a component of his habitual responses to others, resulting in an important reduction of his executive system impairment.

ASSESSMENT: ONGOING, CONTEXTUALIZED, COLLABORATIVE, AND EXPERIMENTAL

Elsewhere we have explained and illustrated an approach to assessment that supports our functional, everyday routine-based approach to intervention (Ylvisaker & Gioia, 1998; Ylvisaker & Feeney, 1998a). In the case of individuals with complex impairment and disability in the domains addressed in this chapter, assessment *for purposes of planning intervention* is ongoing, contextualized, collaborative, and based on careful tests of hypotheses. This approach to assessment has its historical roots in Vygotsky's dynamic assessment (Vygotsky, 1978), elaborated by Feuerstein (1979) and more recently by many practitioners in educational psychology (Palinscar, Brown, & Campione, 1994), special education, speech-language pathology, and other fields. Behavioral psychologists have a long history of assessment by means of experimental analysis of variables that potentially influence behavior (Iwata, Vollmer, & Zarcone, 1990; Kern, Childs, Dunlap, Clarke, & Falk, 1994). This section is restricted to a brief rationale for this type of assessment and an outline of the steps of the assessment.

Rationale

Why Ongoing?

Following severe TBI, individuals can continue spontaneous neurological recovery for months and in some cases years. This by itself mandates ongoing assessment. In addition, changes in environmental and task demands, in the individual's ability levels and psychoreactive responses, and in the skill levels of everyday people in the environment all contribute to unpredictability in evolving outcome, inviting ongoing assessment to ensure that services and supports are maximally effective.

Why Contextualized?

Many neuropsychological studies of people with TBI, or specifically with prefrontal injury, have raised serious questions about the ecological validity of office-bound tests for this group (Benton, 1991; Bigler, 1988; Crépeau, Scherzer, Belleville, & Desmarais, 1997; Dennis, 1991; Dywan and Segalowitz, 1996; Eslinger & Damasio, 1985; Grattan & Eslinger,

1991; Mateer & Williams, 1991; Stelling, McKay, Carr, Walsh, & Bauman, 1986; Stuss & Benson, 1986; Varney & Menefee, 1993; Welsh, Pennington, & Groisser, 1991). Often people with prefrontal injury perform better on standardized tests than one would expect based on real-world performance, because the tests are externally structured and impose few demands in the areas of goal setting, task identification, initiation, self-monitoring, or real-world strategic thinking. Others perform surprisingly poorly on standardized tests because the tasks are novel and the stimulus cues present in the everyday routines of life are not present to support performance. In either case, it is mandatory to make effective use of real-world contexts in functional assessment.

Why Collaborative?

Collaboration increases the number of observations that can be made, the number of real-world contexts that can be explored, and the number of functional experiments that can be performed. In addition, when many people collaborate in assessment, the likelihood is increased that these same people will collaborate in implementing the intervention plan that results from the assessment. Finally, participation in collaborative assessment is an ideal way for everyday people to learn about the realities associated with the disability.

Why Tests of Hypotheses?

All behavior is determined by multiple factors. If a person has trouble with a task, there are typically scores of potential explanations for that difficulty. Similarly, when a person succeeds, that success may be a product of varied strategies. If specialists in rehabilitation do not know why people succeed when they succeed or what underlying impairment explains failure, they are not in a position to create a meaningful, appropriately targeted intervention program. Therefore, alternative hypotheses must be tested.

Assessment Process

Collaboratively Identify the Problem

In some cases, such as the case of Jay described later in this chapter, there is little difficulty identifying the functional problem that calls out for intervention. In other cases, it is not so easy. For example, one and the same issue may be identified by one person as defiance, by another as withdrawal, and by others as lack of initiation or laziness. In these cases, it is critical to agree to a neutral description of the problem behavior before proceeding.

Collaboratively Formulate Hypotheses

Hypotheses may be derived from neurodiagnostic information, from neuropsychological or other testing, from clinical experience with similar individuals, or from real-world interaction with the person whose intervention plan is being developed. Typically, teams of professionals and others have little difficulty generating possible explanations for the person's behavior or proposing intervention plans. It may not be as easy to label one's favored explanation a hypothesis and subject it to testing along with other hypotheses. However, this is precisely the process that enables teams to move beyond conflict over treatment plans and to identify interventions that have a demonstrable effect.

Collaboratively Select Hypotheses To Test

Some hypotheses may be easier to test than others; some may have greater face validity than others; some may have more interesting implications for intervention than others; some may be embraced by more members of the team than others. Selecting hypotheses to test and the order in which to test them requires balancing these considerations.

Collaboratively Test Hypotheses

Exhibit 5–4 illustrates hypothesis-testing assessment by presenting three quite different assessment questions, hypotheses that might be formulated in relation to the questions, proposed tests of the hypotheses, and likely intervention strategies in the event that a given experiment confirms the hypothesis. In some cases, several hypotheses can be tested within a short period of time and possibly within a controlled assessment setting. In other cases, the process extends for weeks and mandates exploration in several real-world settings. In some cases, hypothesis testing is designed to explore the impact of hypothesized variables one at a time. In other cases

Exhibit 5–4 Illustrations of Contextualized, Collaborative Hypothesis Testing

ASSESSMENT QUESTION 1

Question

Why is it that John seems to understand information when I present it to him, but he rarely can state the next day what he has learned? What should we do about this?

Collaborative Hypothesis Generation

John's problem could be a consequence of many cognitive or executive system breakdowns, or combinations of them. For example:

1. *Retrieval:* John processes, encodes, and stores the information, but has difficulty retrieving it the next day.
2. *Storage:* He encodes the information but simply does not retain it.
3. *Organization/encoding:* His initial processing of the information is superficial, making it possible for him to answer questions immediately but not retain the information.
4. *Attention:* He can remember information, but only when he is not distracted at the time of encoding and at the time of retrieval.
5. *Repetition:* He can remember information, but only if it is repeated many times.

Collaborative Hypothesis Testing

Hypothesis 1: Retrieval

John processes, encodes, and stores the information, but has difficulty retrieving it the next day.

Test

Systematically compare John's performance on *free recall* tasks (e.g., "Tell me about the story we read yesterday") versus *recognition memory* tasks (e.g., true/false questions). If John does much better on recognition memory tasks, teachers and others will need to use such tasks in assessing his retention of information.

Hypothesis 2: Storage

John encodes the information, but simply does not retain it.

continues

Exhibit 5–4 continued

Test

Systematically compare John's performance on immediate-recall tasks versus delayed-recall tasks. Vary the time delay. If storage is specifically impaired, John will need memory prostheses.

Hypothesis 3: Organization/Encoding

John's initial processing of the information is superficial, making it possible for him to answer questions immediately but not retain the information.

Test

Systematically compare John's performance on memory tasks when given advance organizers versus no advance organizers. If organizers make a substantial difference, he may benefit from a rich assortment of advance organizers for tasks throughout the day.

Hypothesis 4: Attention

John can remember information, but only when he is not distracted at the time of encoding and at the time of retrieval.

Test

Systematically compare John's performance in the presence of distractions versus no distractions. If distractions substantially impair performance, he may need to receive instruction in a nondistracting environment.

Hypothesis 5: Repetition

John can remember information, but only if it is repeated many times.

Test

Systematically compare John's performance when given only one or two repetitions versus many repetitions. If repetition makes a substantial difference, staff and family will need to find a way to encourage large amounts of repetition.

continues

Exhibit 5–4 continued

ASSESSMENT QUESTION 2

Question

Why does Bill refuse and become aggressive when asked to leave the bus in the morning upon its arrival at school?

Collaborative Hypothesis Generation

Bill's oppositional and aggressive behavior could be the result of many factors. For example:

1. *Confusion:* He may be confused and disoriented when he arrives at school and therefore act out as a result of associated anxiety.
2. *Avoidance:* He may use aggressive behavior to communicate his need or desire to escape nonpreferred activities at school.
3. *Attention:* He may act out because he enjoys the attention that he routinely gets from many staff members and other students when he is acting out.

Collaborative Hypothesis Testing

Hypothesis 1: Confusion

Because of significant cognitive and organizational impairments, Bill does not understand what is happening and is afraid.

Test

Compare the frequency, intensity, and duration of challenging behavior with no preparation for the bus-to-school transition versus when the bus-to-school transitional routine includes preparation using photographs of school staff and school activities and consistent orientation to the first activity of the day, given while Bill is still on the bus, and a routine welcome from school staff before Bill leaves the bus.

Hypothesis 2: Avoidance

Bill does not like the activities that are expected of him when he arrives at school and he successfully avoids these nonpreferred activities by engaging in challenging behaviors.

continues

Exhibit 5–4 continued

Test

Compare the frequency, intensity, and duration of challenging behavior with no change in the current routine versus (1) when Bill is given the opportunity to choose the first activities of the day and (2) when activities are systematically altered (such as one week of math [nonpreferred] upon arrival, then one week of physical education [preferred], then one week of English [nonpreferred]).

Hypothesis 3: Attention

Bill engages in these problem behaviors because he enjoys the attention that he gets from staff and other students when he is acting out.

Test

Compare the frequency, intensity, and duration of challenging behavior with no change in the current routine versus the following experimental alternative routines:

- Wait to ask Bill to leave the bus until all the other students are gone and minimize the number of people who are in proximity to Bill during the bus transition time (testing proximity attention).
- Verbally prompt Bill at the beginning of the bus transition time and then keep verbal interactions at a minimum and only speak in a low voice tone (testing verbal attention).
- Verbally prompt Bill at the beginning of the bus transition time and only speak in a low tone of voice (testing emotional attention).
- Increase the frequency of attention that Bill receives while riding the bus (before the transition) and after entering the school and engaging in prescribed activities.

ASSESSMENT QUESTION 3

Question

Why does Charlie, who was pretraumatically obese, continually ask for food and become aggressive when his requests are denied?

Collaborative Hypothesis Generation

Charlie's uncontrolled eating behavior may be (1) a result of an unknown metabolic or other medical condition, (2) an expression of access-motivated behavior, (3) an expression of his need to control others' behavior.

continues

Exhibit 5–4 continued

Collaborative Hypothesis Testing

Hypothesis 1: Medical

Charlie has an unknown metabolic or medical condition that results in an irresistible drive to eat, which cannot be redirected.

Test

Charlie could be referred for a medical evaluation, including neurology, endocrinology, and gastroenterology consults. If there are positive findings, recommended changes will be made in his program, carefully comparing eating behaviors before and after the change in regimen.

Hypothesis 2: Acquisition

Charlie simply wants to eat and he does whatever it takes to get food.

Test

Compare the frequency and onset of eating-related behaviors under the following conditions:

- Continue with the current attempts to prevent Charlie from getting food.
- For an agreed-upon period of time give Charlie free access to as much food as he would like to eat.

Hypothesis 3: Control

Charlie has few opportunities to control even the most basic elements of his daily routine. The only thing he can really control is what he eats, and he fiercely resists any attempts to control this part of his life.

Test

Compare the frequency and onset of eating-related behaviors under the following conditions:

- Develop a system in which Charlie is able to make decisions about what activities he will engage in and when he will engage in them, including what he will eat and when he will eat it (within agreed-upon limits).
- Use the same system, but have the staff make the decisions about what he will do and when he will do it, including eating.

Source: Reprinted with permission from M. Ylvisaker and T. Feeney, *Collaborative Brain Injury Intervention: Positive Everyday Routines*, © 1998, Singular Publishing Group.

in which the issue to be explored is serious (such as aggressive behavior), requiring immediate attention, it may be desirable to combine hypotheses—that is, experiment with a multifaceted intervention. If the complex hypothesis is confirmed (the intervention is successful), it may not be possible to know which individual hypotheses were confirmed and in what combination, but at least the clinical problem is solved. Feeney and Ylvisaker (1995) presented three single-subject experimental designs that fit this description.

Collaboratively Interpret the Results and Formulate an Intervention Plan

In many cases, the test is a trial intervention. If the trial intervention works well, then the treatment plan may follow in a relatively automatic manner. This proved to be the case with Jay. In other cases, such as Tom (described later in this chapter), the treatment plan was an elaboration of the initial experiments that confirmed the executive system hypothesis. When people have chronic disability in executive system, cognitive, communication, and behavioral domains, intervention often takes the form of supportive modifications of everyday routines, modifications that were identified as positive by means of hypothesis testing (Ylvisaker & Feeney, 1998a).

PROGRESSION OF INTERVENTION

Exhibit 5–5 proposes an understanding of functional intervention that progresses through five critical steps. First, staff and everyday people (ideally including the person with disability) collaborate to identify what is and is not working in the everyday routines of life. For example, in Jay's case (described below) it was clear that his interactive routines with people who irritated him were not working; Jay lost control of himself in response to social provocation and often perseverated on his negative emotionality, frequently losing an entire day of program activities. Tom (described below) was so inattentive in class that he completed few tasks, learned little, and therefore received considerable disapproval from teaching staff.

Second, specialists, everyday people, and if possible the person with disability collaborate to identify what changes in everyday routines could result quickly in reduction of handicap and in the longer run result in

Exhibit 5–5 Progression of Intervention within a Functional, Everyday Approach to Rehabilitation

Step 1:	Identify what is working and what is not working for the individual in everyday routines.
Step 2:	Identify what changes—including changes in the environment, in the behavior of others, and in the individual's own behavior—hold the potential to transform negative, unsuccessful routines into positive, successful routines and build repertoires of positive behavior.
Step 3:	Identify how those changes in everyday routines can become motivating for the individual and for critical everyday people in that environment.
Step 4:	Implement whatever supports are necessary for intensive practice of positive routines in real-world contexts.
Step 5:	Systematically withdraw supports and expand contexts as it becomes possible to do so.

reduction of disability and impairment. In some cases, it is not difficult to identify these changes. For example, everybody agreed that Jay and others in his environment would benefit greatly from his successfully disregarding sources of irritation. However, in other cases, such as Tom's, systematic hypothesis testing (described in the previous section) is required to identify the source of the manifest problem and therefore to identify the most useful and positive changes in everyday routines.

Third, staff, everyday people, and the person with disability collaborate to identify the supports needed for positive changes in everyday routines and ways to motivate these changes for the person with disability and for others in the environment. Often this stage requires considerable creativity and flexibility. There exists no rehabilitation textbook or workbook that can prescribe the unique combinations of supports that are often needed in real-world contexts or that can show how these changes in everyday routine can become palatable and motivating for everyone involved. At this stage, art, creativity, and savvy are more critical than science and book learning.

Fourth, staff, everyday people, and the person with disability collaborate to put systems of support in place so that everyday routines are positive and successful. Jay required well-timed reminders, but reminders framed in language that he had dictated. Tom used an elaborate system of supports that included a consistent, written executive function routine that was detailed and concrete; if possible, graphic advance organizers for any complex or long task; and peer support.

Fifth, staff, everyday people, and the person with disability collaborate to systematically reduce the level of support provided. Of course, good judgment must be exercised. In Tom's case, supports were suddenly removed (because of administrative mistakes) and he regressed to preintervention levels of functioning. In Jay's case, in contrast, the supports were gradually reduced, and a year after the initiation of the intervention he proudly (and correctly) declared that what had been the source of extreme disability and handicap for him (his inability to cope with stressful social interaction) was no longer a problem.

CASE ILLUSTRATIONS

Jay: An Adult with Chronic Executive Function and Associated Impairments

As a teenager, Jay joined the marines and served in the Vietnam war. Following discharge from the marines (with a diagnosis of posttraumatic stress disorder), he earned his graduate equivalency diploma and worked for several years as a cross-country truck driver. In recent years, he has had little contact with his family.

Jay incurred a severe closed head injury in an automobile crash in 1975. Unfortunately, his medical records are unhelpful in identifying the specific location of primary brain injury. Impairment associated with the brain injury includes spastic quadriparesis (he is unable to walk and requires maximal one-person support to transfer), dysarthria (his speech is minimally intelligible to an unfamiliar listener), and executive system impairment (resulting in significant social disinhibition and weakness in anger control, among other disabilities).

In 1997, 22 years after the injury, we began to work with Jay and the staff who served him in a vocational day program. At that time, he lived in a nursing home because no opportunities to live in the community had been offered to him for the previous seven years. Providers of supported living services did not consider Jay a candidate for transfer to a group home, supported apartment, or other less-restrictive living situation because of the frequency of his uncontrolled behavioral outbursts. His two primary goals in the day program were (1) to achieve sufficient control over his communication and behavior that he could live in a nonrestrictive setting of his choice, and (2) to increase the amount of time he spent in productive supported work.

Jay's responses to comments from peers whom he considered disrespectful and to commands, suggestions, and reminders from staff often included obscene gestures; verbally aggressive attacks laced with serious expletives; and attempts to punch, choke, and push others. Although he had been served in the day program for several years, he continued to exhibit opposition to authority figures and severe rigidity in relation to schedule changes. Staff said that they had little control over Jay. They hoped that he would arrive at the program in a good mood and choose to do what he was scheduled to do; if not, staff had no consistently successful strategies to modify or control his behavior. Redirection sometimes worked when Jay was mildly irritated, but only when the redirection was delivered by a favored staff member. However, when Jay was out of control, staff felt they had no option but to push his wheelchair into an empty room (ineffectively instructing him to calm down) where he often continued to yell and punch and kick the wall for several minutes before regaining some control.

The Intervention

Step 1: What Is Working and What Is Not Working in Everyday Routines? The above description of Jay's challenging behavior indicates the primary obstacles to his achieving his goals. His apparent lack of self-control over his reactions to others and over his own internal states rendered him an apparent victim of the whims of his emotional states and of the goodwill and interactive competencies of people in his environment. Unfortunately, his problem had been labeled "behavioral," and staff who served him were accustomed to serving people with behavior problems by creating intervention programs structured around consequences of behavior. Therefore, his days were filled with routines that began with (1) peer or staff provocation (such as a peer laughing at Jay), followed by (2) Jay's angry verbal or gestural response, followed by (3) a staff verbal cue (e.g., "Jay, that's not acceptable") or attempt at redirection, followed often by (4) Jay's steady escalation, followed by (5) staff removing him to an empty room. The shortcomings inherent in consequence-oriented behavior management for people with frontal lobe injury have been explained elsewhere (Feeney & Ylvisaker, 1997; Ylvisaker & Feeney, 1996, 1998a). The neuropsychological literature offers at least three distinct explanations for inefficient learning from consequences in people with frontal lobe injury (Alderman, 1996; Damasio, 1994; Rolls, Hornack, Wade, & McGrath, 1994). The bottom line in this case is that Jay was not getting better and was increasingly feeling a lack of control over his behavior.

Step 2: What Changes—Including Changes in the Environment, in the Behavior of Others, and in the Individual's Own Behavior—Hold the Potential to Transform Negative, Unsuccessful Routines into Positive, Successful Routines and Build Repertoires of Positive Behavior? It was clear to everybody (including Jay when he was calm) that he and staff would both benefit enormously if he could simply ignore the comments, laughter, schedule changes, and other behaviors that provoked him. The hypothesis was that Jay could learn to control his reactions to others, but initially would need to be reminded at exactly the right time that by reacting in an out-of-control manner, he was actually allowing others to control him—which was precisely what he was so passionately opposed to.

Step 3: How Can Positive Changes in Everyday Routines Become Motivating for the Individual and for Critical Everyday People in That Environment? Sensitive to Jay's understanding of himself as a truck driver; as a tough, no-nonsense male adult; and as a person who would not be intimidated or controlled by others, we negotiated with him a system of supportive reminders. The spirit of the negotiation was this: "Jay, you're a strong guy; you're a winner. But when you go ballistic in response to the other guys here, you make them winners—you let them get to you. I don't think you want to do that. What kind of reminder could we give you so you remember that you're the winner; you're the man—not them?" In this negotiation, Jay chose a small number of scripted sentences and phrases (such as "I will spare his life; it's not worth it") to be used by staff as part of an antecedent-focused approach to his poorly controlled behavior. Jay formally authorized staff to whisper one of these scripted utterances in his ear immediately following a provocation by some other person and before Jay responded angrily. Staff were motivated to try the new intervention because they were frustrated with the failure of previous intervention strategies and genuinely wanted to help Jay.

Step 4: What Supports Are Necessary To Ensure Intensive Practice of Positive Routines in Real-World Contexts? Following this negotiation and with Jay's approval, staff then implemented this system of antecedent supports designed to reduce the frequency of Jay's negative behavior and ultimately improve his self-regulation of communication and behavior. Instead of reacting to Jay's behavior, staff now had an anticipatory script that they hoped would ultimately become Jay's own internal script. For several weeks, staff and Jay worked together to create routines such as the following:

Jay: (Is doing his work or conversing.)
Peer: (Makes a joking or derogatory comment interpreted by Jay as provoking.)
Jay: (Begins to tense as a first step in an angry response—clenching his fists.)
Staff: Whispers in Jay's ear: "I'm not going to let him get to me; I will spare his life. If I let him piss me off, he'll win. I'm the winner. It's not worth it."
Jay: Mutters quietly, "Screw him."
Staff: "Awright! You are the man!"

Over the next few months, several hundred of these routines were implemented in the context of the everyday routines of Jay's life, in varied settings and with varied communication partners. Several staff were involved, including a young female speech-language pathology intern who was initially somewhat taken aback that this was her job, but who nevertheless implemented the scripts perfectly.

At the same time, more basic changes were implemented in the daily routines within the program, including executive function routines at the beginning and end of the day. The morning routine included negotiation of daily goals, plans to achieve the goals, and a prediction of success. In addition, Jay was responsible for identifying his "mind set" (his internal state of agitation or of self-control) and for determining what sorts of special supports, if any, he might need to succeed in meeting his goals. Jay's day ended with a self-rating of his performance, a calm review of what worked and what did not work for him over the course of the day, and an identification of the strategies that were particularly helpful. This review helped Jay internalize the positive scripts that staff were using in their attempt to help him control angry outbursts.

Step 5: How Can Supports Be Systematically Withdrawn? After several weeks of systematic cueing and regular reviews of what was working and what was not working, staff and Jay agreed that they could begin to withhold the external cues, or use them only when it appeared (or when Jay said) that he was having a particularly hard time. Jay was largely responsible for this self-assessment (although initially some negotiation with staff was required). For example, if Jay's assessment of his mental state during the morning planning session indicated a need for considerable support, then staff provided more antecedent supports than on other days. In this sense, Jay dictated the schedule of fading of the supports. Cuing was gradually decreased in frequency and in kind (from modeled self-talk to a subtle gestural cue), but not on a rigid schedule. Furthermore, Jay increasingly took responsibility for the afternoon review of his day. He was genuinely interested in his performance in relation to the goals that he had set for himself and proud of his growing self-control. Over the course of this year of treatment, he also began to construct daily goals that were meaningful and consistent with his abilities and needs.

Outcome

Prior to the implementation of the intervention, staff reported that Jay lost an average of two days per week to serious angry outbursts and the prolonged negative emotionality that followed. In addition, several reports of physical attacks on staff and peers in the program had been recorded over the previous year. Since the implementation of the program (one year prior to this writing), no incident reports have been filed and the frequency of wholly nonproductive days has decreased from an average of approximately two days per week to no more than one per month. Significantly, Jay's average amount of productive work time in his day program has increased from approximately 15 minutes per day to three hours per day. These changes have reduced Jay's general levels of frustration and, at the same time, have increased the willingness of staff and peers to interact with him.

In addition, Jay has been offered two opportunities for community residential placement. However, he has not yet accepted either of these offers for reasons that are not entirely clear. He may simply be so accustomed to his nursing home residence that the move appears threatening at this time. In any case, the intervention was successful in enabling Jay to achieve his two primary goals in the day program, goals toward which he had made little progress in the previous several years. Furthermore, Jay now enjoys generally positive relationships with several peers and staff in the program and is extremely proud of his success. He recently summarized his achievement over the past year: "I'm in charge. If you let people get to you, they have won. But I know how to put up with their bullshit. They might think they won, but we all know who got the last word in."

In a process clearly described by Vygotsky 60 years ago, repeated contextualized social interaction using negotiated scripts of self-regulation had been internalized to become part of Jay's automatic executive functioning. An externally supported intervention that began as an attempt to decrease Jay's *handicap* (which included restricted living options and minimal opportunities for productive work) gradually evolved into an intervention that reduced his *disability* (as he increasingly assumed responsibility for self-cuing) and finally into an intervention that reduced his *impairment* (as the self-reminders became less deliberate and increasingly part of his automatic executive system).

Tom: A Child with Chronic Executive Function and Associated Impairments

As a young preschooler, Tom had a cerebellar tumor that progressively overgrew his cortical mantel. Treatment included large amounts of intracranial radiation and chemotherapy. Early outcome was characterized by moderate motor, perceptual, and cognitive impairment. With therapy, Tom learned to walk and to speak intelligibly. His cognitive impairment was not debilitating during his preschool years, and his language development was sufficient to enable him to negotiate most everyday social interactions. However, the disability associated with his cognitive impairment grew as the grade school curriculum gradually increased in its cognitive demands. By third grade, resource room support and standard classroom accommodations (such as extra time, materials modified to meet Tom's perceptual needs) were insufficient to meet Tom's educational needs. However, his regular education teacher was devoted to him and made heroic efforts to help him succeed. Unfortunately, his fourth-grade teacher did not approach her job with Tom in the same positive manner as the third-grade teacher. At the same time, there occurred a substantial increase in the demands of the curriculum, particularly with regard to the abstractness of the academic material and the quantity of material to organize and process efficiently (such as comprehending and composing extended written text).

At the end of fourth grade, the teacher recommended strongly that Tom be educated in a self-contained school for children with severe disability. Tom's parents insisted that he continue in a regular education classroom with resource room support and a paraprofessional aide. The next year, Tom's fifth-grade teacher and a resource room special educator in her first year of employment worked hard to help Tom succeed but, by the Christmas break, school staff were close to concluding that Tom was incapable of profiting from his current placement. It was at that time that we were invited to help family and staff create a more effective educational program for Tom.

The Intervention

Step 1: What Is Working and What Is Not Working in Everyday Routines? Clearly, Tom was struggling in school. When given moderately difficult tasks, he would begin his work, get stuck, and then sit, waiting for someone to save him. This job typically fell to his aide, who felt needed because of Tom's dependence on her, but who was becoming increasingly impatient and increasingly convinced that his failure was deliberate. Therefore, their interaction included considerable nagging from her, followed by angry reactions from Tom. On the positive side, Tom approached most tasks enthusiastically, was generally friendly and upbeat, and had friends in the resource room.

Step 2: What Changes—Including Changes in the Environment, in the Behavior of Others, and in the Individual's Own Behavior—Hold the Potential to Transform Negative, Unsuccessful Routines into Positive, Successful Routines and Build Repertoires of Positive Behavior? In Tom's case, answering this question required considerably more effort than in Jay's case. At the first team meeting we attended in January of Tom's fifth-grade year, four distinct hypotheses were offered. The regular education teacher suggested that the problem appeared to be an extreme attentional impairment, so extreme that she feared he might be experiencing ongoing seizures. Tom's aide was convinced that he was becoming lazy and increasingly oppositional. The new special educator tentatively suggested that the core of Tom's problem was slow processing—so slow that she feared he might not be able to profit from the regular educational setting. We suspected that the core of the problem was organizational impairment. In addition, Tom's mother indicated that Tom was able to do more at home than he was reportedly doing at school, suggesting to her that supports at school must be insufficient.

After some discussion, team members agreed that all of these hypotheses were reasonable and supported by some observations. Therefore, hypothesis testing was required. The team agreed to test the organizational hypothesis first, in part because it was fairly easy to test and, if confirmed, would yield a fairly clear direction for intervention and academic support.

The tests were several mini-experiments, including one carried out in the resource room by the special educator. She first instructed Tom to write a summary of a story that he had read in class. She gave him an hour to complete the task and offered no supports. After several minutes, she observed Tom to be quietly staring off into space. He had written three short sentences, had gotten stuck, and had then completely lost focus. After delivering several impatient prompts with no success, she let Tom hand in the summary, which was as disappointing to him as it was to her.

The next day, she gave Tom the same assignment. However, this time, she and Tom worked together to place critical information in a graphic advance organizer so that he would have an organized guide to help him write the summary (Ylvisaker, Szekeres, & Haarbauer-Krupa, 1998). With this organizational support, Tom wrote an adequately elaborated and well-organized summary that was judged to be an excellent product by the teacher and enabled Tom to feel proud of his work. This and several similar experiments convinced staff and parents that at the core of Tom's problem lurked severe impairment of planning and organizing, as well as other related executive functions (e.g., working memory and initiation). His poorly regulated attention and academic failure were judged to be largely secondary to these executive system disturbances.

Because Tom's problem was a general executive system impairment, we chose to frame his organizational support within a larger executive system routine (Ylvisaker, Szekeres, & Feeney, 1998). All of his academic tasks—and some nonacademic tasks—were outlined for him on a form that he called his "task sheet." At the top was a statement of his *Goal* (e.g., complete a workbook page of math problems; write a story); this was followed by his *Plan* (i.e., a task analysis, listing in detailed sequence the steps that he must complete, sometimes in graphic form); toward the bottom of the page were two 1 to 10 rating scales for him and a teacher or aide to rate his performance; finally, there were two columns for his review of his performance, headed "What worked?" and "What didn't work?" These task sheets were all kept in an attractive notebook that Tom called his "Independence Book," so called because he had come to recognize the importance for him of this support in relation to his goal of increased independence.

Step 3: How Can Positive Changes in Everyday Routines Become Motivating for the Individual and for Critical Everyday People in That Environment? Motivation was not a major problem for Tom. The experiments had convinced him, as they had convinced staff, that he needed this kind of support. The problem was rather at the logistical end, identifying who would create the task sheets for all of Tom's tasks—and when. The leadership role fell to the resource room teacher, directing the aide to complete most basic task analyses for Tom. At home, Tom's mother increasingly provided him with advance organizers so that his dependence on her might be lessened. And several weeks after the program was initiated, Tom began to write simple organizers for himself.

Step 4: What Supports Are Necessary To Ensure Intensive Practice of Positive Routines in Real-World Contexts? The keys to the success of Tom's executive function support program were his resource room teacher, who coordinated the program; his aide, who initially filled out most of the task sheets and for the first several weeks of the program cued Tom to use them; and his mother, who used a similar support system at home to facilitate growth in Tom's executive functioning. The executive system routine, with embedded advance organizer, was the focal point of his support system.

Step 5: How Can Supports Be Systematically Withdrawn? One of our roles as consultants was to encourage the resource room teacher to monitor Tom's use of his independence book so that he would experience success, but also so that the paraprofessional's support could be withdrawn as quickly as possible. Tom's aide had been with him for more than two years and was accustomed to using frequent and demanding verbal cues with Tom (often interpreted as nagging). With the special educator's encouragement, the aide increased the time she spent with other children in the classroom and encouraged Tom to ask for her help only when he needed it. By June of that year, Tom was accustomed to looking for a task sheet when he began any new assignment. If he did not find one, he either asked the aide to prepare one for him or (occasionally) he attempted to prepare his own, complete with a task analysis.

Outcome

Table 5–1 presents executive system ratings assigned by Tom's classroom teacher, special educator, and mother in January, when the intervention began, and again in June, at the end of fifth grade. The executive system rating scale is described by Ylvisaker, Szekeres, and Feeney (1998). The dramatic improvements in grade-level ratings in several domains of executive functioning (from kindergarten/first-grade levels in several domains, to fourth-/fifth-grade levels) demonstrate a profound reduction in Tom's handicap. Because of the supports that were put in place for him, he learned more efficiently, was recognized by teachers and others as a contributor and a person with academic potential, and enjoyed the experience of growing independence. Furthermore, by the end of the year, he was beginning to use his external supports without the help of others, suggesting an initial reduction in disability.

Unfortunately, despite a well-written individualized education plan (IEP) and a self-advocacy, transitional videotape that the team helped Tom make so that he could explain the supports he needed to his sixth-grade staff, his program of supports collapsed as he began middle school. School district administrators had neglected to enroll him in the middle school

Table 5–1 Tom's Executive System Ratings

	January, Grade 5			*June, Grade 5*			*October, Grade 6*	
	CT	*SE*	*M*	*CT*	*SE*	*M*	*CT*	*Aide*
Planning/organizing	1	1	1	4	4	4	K	K/1
Initiation	1	K/1	1	4	4	4	K	1/2
Inhibition	K	K/1	3	4	4	5	6	3
General independence	K	K/1	1	5	4/5	4	K	1/2
Orientation to task/ flexibility	1	2	1	5	5	4	K	1
Understanding of task difficulty	K	2	2	3	5	4	K	K/1
Self-monitoring/ Self-evaluating	K	K	2	3	3	4	K	K/1
Strategic behavior	K	2	2	3	5	4	K	K/1

Key: CT = classroom teacher; SE = special educator; M = mother; Aide = paraprofessional classroom aide; numbers refer to grade-level functioning.

Source: Data from M. Ylvisaker, S. Szekeres, and T. Feeney, Cognitive Rehabilitation: Executive Functions in Traumatic Brain Injury Rehabilitation: Children and Adolescents, M. Ylvisaker, ed. © 1998, Butterworth-Heinemann.

resource room and, because it was filled, he had no special education support when the school year began. Furthermore, district administrators had neglected to hire a paraprofessional aide for Tom. Therefore, his year started very badly and his old habits of passivity, lack of initiation, and inattentiveness returned. Clearly his impairment had not been reduced by the previous year's intervention and he needed ongoing executive system supports.

It took the better part of Tom's sixth-grade year to reimplement the program that had demonstrated such benefit for him in fifth grade. Modified versions of the supports continued to be used in seventh and eighth grade, with considerable success as reported by Tom's mother. At the end of eighth grade, Tom passed his state competency exam in reading and came within two points of passing in writing—two subjects in which Tom had no potential for academic growth, according to his fourth-grade teacher. Tom's mother said that he had internalized his routine of requesting modification of his materials (such as size of writing on workbook pages) and organizational support. That is, his earlier habit of simply waiting for somebody to recognize his difficulty and save him was a thing of the distant past. Furthermore, he had become active in initiating interaction with peers and had several friends.

In light of the fact that his fourth-grade teacher had confidently asserted that he had no academic potential, this outcome is positive indeed. Interventions put in place for Tom in fifth grade and continued thereafter (albeit inconsistently and with overly abrupt unplanned reductions and reintroductions of supports) had a marked and undeniable effect in reducing Tom's handicap. In addition, his growing habit of asserting his compensatory needs and using compensatory strategies for important tasks has resulted in a reduction of his academic and social disability. Whereas when he was in fourth grade, specialists predicted growing disability based on the nature and severity of his impairment, in fact his disability was lessened over the next four years by everyday people in his life putting in place supported, everyday routines and then reducing those supports when it became possible to do so.

CONCLUSION

This chapter has presented a functional and highly contextualized approach to rehabilitation for people with TBI whose chronic impairment is in the territory in which cognition, communication, behavior, and executive functions intersect and interact. Both Tom and Jay had *communication impairment*. Jay's was most evident in his aggressive social interaction; Tom's in his passive interactive style and difficulty with organized discourse. Both had *cognitive impairment*. Tom's planning and organizational impairment was pronounced and negatively affected his performance across many contexts in school and elsewhere; Jay had serious difficulty interpreting the behavior of others and monitoring his own. Both had *behavioral impairment*. Jay's behavior problem was of such severity that he was judged incapable of living outside of a highly restrictive nursing home. Although Tom was generally compliant and therefore less likely to wear the label "behavior problem," his low levels of initiation resulted in academic problems. He was also beginning to hit bumpy times with his paraprofessional aide because of the extent of her perceived nagging. Finally, in both cases, as in so many cases following TBI, the core of the problem was *impaired executive functions*—that is, impaired self-regulation of behavior in the pursuit of real-world goals.

In both cases, intervention took the form of reshaping everyday routines, initially to reduce failure and associated academic, social, and vocational handicap. With supports in place—including modifications in the behavior of everyday communication partners—handicap was quickly and dramatically reduced. With massive amounts of contextualized practice in the use of compensatory procedures, both Jay and Tom assumed progressively greater responsibility for their strategic behavior and, therefore, for successful performance—thus reducing their disability. Finally, in both cases, their positive compensatory behaviors became sufficiently routinized that they experienced some degree of reduction of impairment, Jay more than Tom.

With both Jay and Tom, this intervention began many years following onset of problems. We selected these two individuals in part to communicate optimism about the possibility of significant improvement in functioning, even when impairment seems fixed and problems seem intractable and may be worsening. It is important to emphasize that in these two cases—and in many, many others—the problems should not have been allowed to evolve. Alert professionals at any stage of the individual's recovery and of life after the injury could and should have modified everyday routines to prevent the increasing disability and associated handicap.

Economists teach us that the long run is a series of short runs. The same can be said of life after brain injury. From acute rehabilitation; through home, school, job, and community reentry; to outpatient therapies; to evolving supports in school, on the job, or in places of residence, competent professionals can collaborate with people with disability and the everyday people in their lives to create successful everyday routines. At each stage, responsible clinicians focus on the quality and therapeutic value of current routines, on the competencies needed by everyday people in the individual's current contexts of life, and on the preparation needed by the professionals and important everyday people at the next stage (Ylvisaker & Feeney, 1998b). If the baton of clinical wisdom continues to be passed in this manner, the likelihood of functional deterioration over time of the sort experienced by both Tom and Jay is reduced dramatically. And if specialists and everyday people are effective in creating positive, everyday routines of action and interaction, they increase the likelihood of improvements at every level—handicap, disability, and impairment.

Exhibit 5–6 summarizes two fundamentally different approaches to rehabilitation for people with cognitive, communication, behavioral, and executive system impairment. Because intervention possibilities in most of the domains listed in this exhibit exist on a continuum, there are not two, but rather a very large number of meaningful approaches to intervention that could be described using this system of categories. This description of intervention options highlights the choices that are open to clinicians, underscores parallel movements in three apparently distinct disciplines (speech-language pathology, behavioral psychology, and cognitive rehabilitation), and summarizes the components of a functional approach to rehabilitation.

Discussion Questions

1. What are the key differences between intervention that progresses from impairment to disability to handicap, and intervervention that progresses from handicap to disability to impairment?
2. Why should assessment be extended beyond office-bound assessment procedures?
3. Why was it critical for Jay to be involved in choosing the types of support that he needed to overcome his impulsive and aggressive responses to others?
4. What might have been done to prevent the regression that Tom experienced in sixth grade?

Exhibit 5–6 Conventional versus Functional Approaches to Intervention after Brain Injury: Communication, Behavior, and Cognition

SCOPE OF INTERVENTION

Conventional Approach

1. *Speech-language pathology:* The focus is on speech and specific aspects of linguistic competence (semantics, syntax, morphology).
2. *Behavioral psychology:* The focus is on management of specific problem behaviors in a narrow sense.
3. *Cognitive rehabilitation:* The focus is on neuropsychological assessment and intervention that sequentially targets separate components of cognition, arranged in a hierarchy for treatment purposes.

Functional Approach

1. The focus of each profession is on helping individuals with brain injury achieve their real-world goals in real-world contexts, including academic, vocational, and social success.
2. Correctly understood, applied behavior analysis in psychology, pragmatics in speech-language pathology, and social-cognitive intervention in cognitive rehabilitation are essentially the same service, necessitating close collaboration among service providers.
3. Each profession recognizes the overarching importance of executive or self-control functions for academic, vocational, and social success.

INTEGRATION OF INTERVENTION: COLLABORATION

Conventional Approach

1. Cognition, communication, and behavior are targeted for assessment and intervention by separate professionals working in relative isolation.
2. Evaluation reports, including proposed goals, objectives, and plans to achieve the objectives, are produced separately by three professionals.

Functional Approach

1. Although behavioral psychologists, cognitive rehabilitation specialists (including special educators), and speech-language pathologists are recognized as possessing special and unique expertise, the important overlap in their services is frankly acknowledged.
2. Assessments are conducted and plans for intervention are developed in an integrated manner. Ideally, reports are written as integrated, cross-disciplinary documents.

continues

Exhibit 5–6 continued

3. Individuals with disability and significant everyday people in their lives are included as contributing members of the collaborative assessment and intervention teams.

ORIENTATION OF INTERVENTION: DEFICITS AND STRENGTHS

Conventional Approach: Deficit Orientation

1. The *cognitive rehabilitation specialist* attempts to remediate cognitive deficits and restore specific preexisting cognitive skills in areas of impairment.
2. The *speech-language pathologist* attempts to remediate communication deficits and restore specific preexisting speech and language skills in areas of impairment.
3. The *behavioral psychologist* attempts to eliminate undesirable behaviors (such as noncompliance, agitation, combativeness) and increase specific desirable behaviors (such as participation, "socially appropriate" behaviors).

Functional Approach: Strength Orientation

1. Each professional begins with existing strengths and builds upon them with (a) attempts to ensure success in functional activities at the individual's current level of capacity, (b) apprenticeship procedures (including chaining and shaping), and (c) compensatory strategies, using strengths to compensate for weaknesses.
2. Success is a goal throughout intervention, using whatever antecedent supports may be necessary to succeed at functional tasks at the individual's current level of ability.
3. Undesirable and challenging behaviors, including explicitly communicative behaviors, are never simply extinguished without an attempt to substitute a positive alternative that achieves the same goal.
4. Preservation and enhancement of the individual's self-esteem is a background goal for all professionals.

SERVICE DELIVERY: SETTINGS AND ACTIVITIES

Conventional Approach

1. The *speech-language pathologist* uses repetitive drill and practice in isolated settings that bear little resemblance to real-world communica-

continues

Exhibit 5–6 continued

tion settings (such as pull-out therapy). Activities in therapy settings are not necessarily related to real-world communication activities.

2. The *cognitive rehabilitation specialist* uses repetitive drill and practice in isolated settings that bear little resemblance to real-world settings (such as pull-out therapy using decontextualized workbook or computer exercises). Activities in therapy settings are not necessarily related to real-world activities that require the targeted cognitive skill.
3. The *behavioral psychologist* delivers targeted behavioral services on a behavior unit, in a neurobehavioral rehabilitation facility, or in a behavior classroom, with little opportunity to facilitate transfer of training to real-world settings and tasks.

Functional Approach

1. Each profession focuses on real-world needs in real-world contexts. This focus includes supports for achieving real-world goals in real-world contexts and practice of functional communication, social, and cognitive skills in real-world contexts. Specific aspects of the individual's environments and demands in those environments are considered in choosing objectives.
2. As much as possible, communication and behavioral services are delivered in meaningful social groups, in settings that resemble settings in which the skills will need to be used, and in the context of meaningful activities.
3. Pursuit of cognitive, executive function, communication, and behavioral goals is largely in the context of everyday routines, involving modification of those routines with supports that are gradually withdrawn as the individual's skills improve.

PROVIDERS OF SERVICE: INVOLVEMENT OF EVERYDAY COMMUNICATION PARTNERS

Conventional Approach

1. Professionals are considered the primary agents of change in the individual with disability.
2. Each profession focuses primarily on remediation of deficits in the individual; that is, the intervention is impairment oriented.

Functional Approach

1. Each profession focuses on improvement of function within everyday routines. Therefore, everyday communication partners (such as family

continues

Exhibit 5–6 continued

members, paraprofessional aides, supervisors, teachers, coworkers, friends) are critical deliverers of rehabilitation services and supports.

2. A primary role of rehabilitation specialists is to train and provide ongoing supports for everyday communication partners. Within a rehabilitation facility, evening and weekend staff are recognized as particularly critical to the development of a positive and therapeutically efficient rehabilitation environment.

SOURCE OF CONTROL

Conventional Approach

1. There is near total reliance on external control of behavior. Little emphasis is placed on helping the individual to set goals and make good choices, plan how to achieve selected goals, monitor and evaluate behavior in relation to those goals, or make strategic decisions in the face of failure. Professionals assume responsibility for most executive dimensions of behavior.
2. The individual with disability is not included as a member of the team of people who perform assessments, select goals and objectives, plan intervention, monitor and evaluate performance, and create strategic solutions to problems as they arise over the course of intervention.

Functional Approach

1. The ultimate goal is to ensure that the individual controls his or her behavior as much as possible by means of effective decision making, strategic thinking, self-regulation of behavior, and self-regulated control over environmental contingencies.
2. The individual with disability is included as a member of the team of people who perform assessments, select goals and objectives, plan intervention, monitor and evaluate performance, and create strategic solutions to problems as they arise over the course of intervention.

INTERVENTION PROCEDURES

Conventional Approach

1. Prescriptive behavioral objectives specify isolated targets; for example, specific language behaviors are selected for training.
2. Modification of behavior is largely a result of the manipulation of the *consequences* of behavior. Within training tasks, correct performance

continues

Exhibit 5–6 continued

of the target behavior is consequated with presumably desirable objects or events; failure to use the target behavior is followed by a withholding of rewards, a cost of some kind, removal from the situation, or some other neutral or undesirable consequence.

Functional Approach

1. The goal is an acceptable *range* of behaviors (versus a specific behavior) that may vary in their effectiveness in achieving the communicative objective.
2. Modification of behavior (including cognitive and social behavior) is considered a result of manipulating the consequences as well as antecedents of the behavior, but the focus is on *antecedents*. Antecedent control procedures include creating environmental supports; avoiding triggers for negative behavior; inducing positive setting events; generating positive momentum; creating opportunities for choice and control; establishing familiar, positive routines and effective procedures for deviating from routines; providing advance organizers for difficult tasks; teaching scripts for negotiating difficult social situations; and ensuring that the individual has maximal self-management skills.
3. Contingency management (that is, manipulation of consequences of behavior) focuses on positive consequences for desirable behavior (versus punishing consequences and "time out" for negative behavior) and on natural contingencies (versus artificial rewards).
    - As much as possible, rewards are internally related to the action performed. For example, when people request something appropriately, they get it; when people initiate social interaction, they are rewarded with a pleasant interaction; when people use strategies, they succeed in their endeavors.
    - Feedback (positive or negative) is given as much as possible by natural communication partners (such as peers or family members).
4. As much as possible, teaching and learning take place within an apprenticeship relationship. The teacher and the learner are jointly engaged in projects designed to achieve meaningful goals. Initially, the teacher assumes much of the responsibility for achieving the goal, but turns over responsibility to the learner/apprentice as soon as possible.

Source: Reprinted with permission from M. Ylvisaker and T. Feeney, *Collaborative Brain Injury Intervention: Positive Everyday Routines*, © 1998, Singular Publishing Group.

REFERENCES

Adams, J.H., Graham, D.I., Scott, G., Parker, L.S., & Doyle, D. (1980). Brain damage in fatal non-missle head injury. *Journal of Clinical Pathology*, *33*, 1132–1145.

Alderman, N. (1996). Central executive deficit and response to operant conditioning methods. *Neuropsychological Rehabilitation*, *6*, 161–186.

Benton, A. (1991). Prefrontal injury and behavior in children. *Developmental Neuropsychology*, *7*, 275–281.

Biddle, K.R., McCabe, A., & Bliss, L.S. (1996). Narrative skills following traumatic brain injury in children and adults. *Journal of Communication Disorders*, *29*, 447–470.

Bigler, E.D. (1988). Frontal lobe damage and neuropsychological assessment. *Archives of Clinical Neuropsychology*, *3*, 279–297.

Carr, E.G., Levin, L., McConnachie, G., Carlson, J.I., Kemp, D.C., & Smith, C.E. (1994). *Communication-based intervention for problem behavior: A user's guide for producing positive change*. Baltimore: Paul H. Brookes Publishing.

Carr, E.G., Reeve, C.E., Magito-McLaughlin, D. (1997). Contextual influences on problem behavior in people with developmental disabilities. In L.K. Koegel, R.L. Koegel, & G. Dunlap (Eds.), *Positive behavioral support: Including people with difficult behavior in the community* (pp. 403–423). Baltimore: Paul H. Brookes Publishing.

Chapman, S.B. (1997). Cognitive-communication abilities in children with closed head injury. *American Journal of Speech-Language Pathology*, *6*, 50–58.

Chapman, S.B., Levin, H.S., Matejka, J., Harward, H.N., & Kufera, J. (1995). Discourse ability in head injured children: Consideration of linguistic, psychosocial, and cognitive factors. *Journal of Head Trauma Rehabilitation*, *10*, 36–54.

Chapman, S.B., Watkins, R., Gustafson, C., Moore, S., Levin, H.S., & Kufera, J.A. (1997). Narrative discourse in children with closed head injury, children with language impairment, and typically developing children. *American Journal of Speech-Language Pathology*, *6*, 66–76.

Crépeau, F., Scherzer, B.P., Belleville, S., & Desmarais, G. (1997). A qualitative analysis of central executive disorders in a real-life work situation. *Neuropsychological Rehabilitation*, *7*, 147–165.

Damasio, A.R. (1994). *Descartes' error*. New York: Avon Books.

Dennis, M. (1991). Frontal lobe function in childhood and adolescence: A heuristic for assessing attention regulation, executive control, and the intentional states important for social discourse. *Developmental Neuropsychology*, *7*, 327–358.

Dennis, M. (1992). Word-finding in children and adolescents with a history of brain injury. *Topics in Language Disorders*, *13*, 66–82.

Dennis, M., & Barnes, M. (1990). Knowing the meaning, getting the point, bridging the gap, and carrying the message: Aspects of discourse following closed head injury in childhood and adolescence. *Brain and Language*, *39*, 428–446.

Dennis, M., Barnes, M.A., Donnelly, R.E., Wilkinson, M., & Humphreys, R.P. (1996). Appraising and managing knowledge: Metacognitive skills after childhood head injury. *Developmental Neuropsychology*, *12*, 77–103.

Dennis, M., & Lovett, M. (1990). Discourse ability in children after brain damage. In Y. Joanette & H.H. Brownell (Eds.), *Discourse ability and brain damage: Theoretical and empirical perspectives* (pp. 199–223). New York: Springer-Verlag.

Dywan, J., & Segalowitz, S.J. (1996). Self- and family ratings of adaptive behavior after traumatic brain injury: Psychometric scores and frontally generated RRPs. *Journal of Head Trauma Rehabilitation, 11*, 79–75.

Eslinger, P.J., & Damasio, A.R. (1985). Severe disturbance of higher cognition following bilateral frontal lobe oblation: Patient EVR. *Neurology, 35*, 1731–1741.

Feeney, T.J., & Ylvisaker, M. (1995). Choice and routine: Antecedent behavioral interventions for adolescents with severe traumatic brain injury. *Journal of Head Trauma Rehabilitation, 10*, 67–86.

Feeney, T.J., & Ylvisaker, M. (1997). A positive, communication-based approach to challenging behavior after TBI. In A. Glang, G.H.S. Singer, & B. Todis (Eds.), *Children with acquired brain injury: The school's response* (pp. 229–254). Baltimore: Paul H. Brookes Publishing.

Feuerstein, R. (1979). *The dynamic assessment of retarded performers: The learning potential assessment device: Theory, instruments, and techniques*. Baltimore: University Park Press.

Fey, M. (1986). *Language intervention with young children*. San Diego: College-Hill Press.

Finset, A., & Andresen, S. (1990). The process diary concept: An approach in training orientation, memory and behaviour control. In R.L. Wood & I. Fussey (Eds.), *Cognitive rehabilitation in perspective* (pp. 99–116). London: Taylor & Francis Publishers.

Giangreco, M.F., Cloninger, C.J., & Iverson, V.S. (1993). *Choosing options and accommodations for children (COACH): A guide to planning inclusive education*. Baltimore: Paul H. Brookes Publishing.

Grattan, L.M., & Eslinger, P.J. (1991). Frontal lobe damage in children and adults: A comparative review. *Developmental Neuropsychology, 7*, 283–326.

Groher, M. (1990). Communication disorders in adults. In M. Rosenthal, E. Griffith, M. Bond, & J.D. Miller (Eds.), *Rehabilitation of the adult and child with traumatic brain injury* (pp. 148–162). Philadelphia: F.A. Davis.

Hagen, C. (1981). Language disorders secondary to closed head injury. *Topics in Language Disorders, 1*, 73–87.

Hartley, L.L. (1995). *Cognitive-communicative abilities following brain injury: A functional approach*. San Diego, CA: Singular Publishing Group.

Horner, R.H., Dunlap, G., & Koegel, R.L. (Eds.). (1988). *Generalization and maintenance: Lifestyle changes in applied settings*. Baltimore: Paul H. Brookes Publishing.

Iwata, B.A., Vollmer, T.R., & Zarcone, J.R. (1990). The experimental (functional) analysis of behavior disorders: Methodology, applications, and limitations. In A.C. Repp & N.N. Singh (Eds.), *Perspectives on the use of nonaversive and aversive interventions for persons with developmental disabilities* (pp. 301–330). Sycamore, IL: Sycamore Publishing Co.

Kennedy, C.H. (1994). Manipulating antecedent conditions to alter the stimulus control of problem behavior. *Journal of Applied Behavior Analysis, 27*, 161–170.

Kern, L., Childs, K.E., Dunlap, G., Clarke, S., & Falk, G.D. (1994). Using assessment based curricular intervention to improve the classroom behavior of a student with emotional and behavioral challenges. *Journal of Applied Behavior Analysis*, *27*, 7–19.

Koegel, R., & Koegel, L.K. (1995). *Teaching children with autism: Strategies for initiating positive interactions and improving learning opportunities*. Baltimore: Paul H. Brookes Publishing.

Koegel, L.K., Koegel R.L., & Dunlap G. (1997). *Positive behavioral support: Including people with difficult behavior in the community*. Baltimore: Paul H. Brooks Publishing.

Levin, H.S., Goldstein, F.C., Williams, D.H., & Eisenberg, H.M. (1991). The contribution of frontal lobe lesions to the neurobehavioral outcome of closed head injury. In H.S. Levin, H.M. Eisenberg, & A.L. Benton (Eds.), *Frontal lobe function and dysfunction* (pp. 318–338). New York: Oxford University Press.

Liles, B.J., Coelho, C.A., Duffy, R.J., & Zalagens, M.R. (1989). Effects of elicitation procedures on the narratives of normal and closed head-injured adults. *Journal of Speech and Hearing Disorders*, *54*, 356–366.

MacDonald, J. (1989). *Becoming partners with children: From play to conversation*. Chicago: Riverside Publishing Co.

Martin, G., & Pear, J. (1996). *Behavior modification: What it is and how to do it* (5th ed.). Upper Saddle River, NJ: Prentice Hall.

Mateer, C.A., & Williams, D. (1991). Effects of frontal lobe injury in childhood. *Developmental Neuropsychology*, *7*, 359–376.

McDonald, S. (1992a). Communication disorders following closed head injury: New approaches to assessment and rehabilitation. *Brain Injury*, *6*, 283–292.

McDonald, S. (1992b). Differential pragmatic language loss following severe closed head injury: Inability to comprehend conversational implicature. *Applied Psycholinguistics*, *13*, 295–312.

McDonald, S. (1993). Pragmatic language skills after closed head injury: Ability to meet the informational needs of the listener. *Brain and Language*, *44*, 28–46.

Mendelsohn, D., Levin, H.S., Bruce, D., Lilly, M.A., Harward, H., Culhane, K., & Eisenberg, H.M. (1992). Late MRI after head injury in children: Relationship to clinical features and outcome. *Child's Nervous System*, *8*, 445–452.

Mentis, M., & Prutting, C.A. (1991). Analysis of topic as illustrated in a head-injured and a normal adult. *Journal of Speech and Hearing Research*, *34*, 583–595.

Morris, E.K. (1992). The aim, progress, and evolution of behavior analysis. *The Behavior Analyst*, *15*, 3–29.

Palinscar, A.S., Brown, A.L., & Campione, J.C. (1994). Models and practices of dynamic assessment. In G.P. Wallach & K.G. Butler (Eds.), *Language-learning disabilities in school-age children and adolescents* (pp. 132–144). New York: McMillan.

Ponsford, J. (1990). The use of computers in the rehabilitation of attention disorders. In R.L. Wood & I. Fussey (Eds.), *Cognitive rehabilitation in perspective* (pp. 48–67). London: Taylor & Francis Publishers.

Pressley, M. (1995). More about the development of self-regulation: Complex, long-term, and thoroughly social. *Educational Psychology*, *30*, 207–212.

Reichle, J., & Wacker, D.P. (Eds.). (1993). *Communicative alternatives to challenging behavior*. Baltimore: Paul H. Brookes Publishing.

Rolls, E.T., Hornack, J., Wade, D., & McGrath, J. (1994). Emotion-related learning in patients with social and emotional changes associated with frontal lobe damage. *Journal of Neurology, Neurosurgery, and Psychiatry*, *57*, 1518–1524.

Ruff, R.M., Baser, C.A., Johnston, J.W., Marshall, L.F., Klauber, S.K., Klauber, M.R., & Minteer, M. (1989). Neuropsychological rehabilitation: An experimental study with head-injured patients. *Journal of Head Trauma Rehabilitation*, *4*, 20–36.

Sarno, M.T., Buonaguro, A., & Levita, E. (1986). Characteristics of verbal impairment in closed head injured patients. *Archives of Physical Medicine and Rehabilitation*, *67*, 400–405.

Schacter, D.L., & Glisky, E.L. (1986). Memory remediation: Restoration, alleviation, and the acquisition of domain-specific knowledge. In B. Uzzell & Y. Gross (Eds.), *Clinical neuropsychology of intervention* (pp. 257–282). Boston: Martinus Nijhoff.

Singley, M.K., & Anderson, J.R. (1989). *Transfer of cognitive skill*. Cambridge, MA: Harvard University Press.

Sohlberg, M., & Mateer, C. (1989). *Introduction to cognitive rehabilitation: Theory and practice*. New York: Guilford Press.

Stelling, M.W., McKay, S.E., Carr, W.A., Walsh, J.W., & Bauman, R.J. (1986). Frontal lobe lesions and cognitive function in craniopharyngioma survivors. *American Journal of Diseases of Childhood*, *140*, 710–714.

Stuss, D.T., & Benson, D.F. (1986). *The frontal lobes*. New York: Raven Press.

Turkstra, L.S., & Holland, A.L. (1998). Assessment of syntax after adolescent brain injury: Effects of memory on test performance. *Journal of Speech, Language, and Hearing Research*, *41*, 137–149.

Varney, N.R., & Menefee, L. (1993). Psychosocial and executive deficits following closed head injury: Implications for orbital frontal cortex. *Journal of Head Trauma Rehabilitation*, *8*, 32–44.

von Cramon, D.Y., & Matthes-von Cramon, G. (1994). Back to work with a chronic dysexecutive syndrome? (A case report). *Neuropsychological Rehabilitation*, *4*, 399–417.

Vygotsky, L.S. (1978). *Mind in society: The development of higher psychological processes* (M. Cole, V. John-Steiner, S. Scribner, & E. Souberman, Eds. & Trans.). Cambridge, MA: Harvard University Press.

Vygotsky, L.S. (1981). The genesis of higher mental functions. In J.V. Wertsch (Ed.), *The concept of activity in Soviet psychology* (pp. 144–189). Armonk, NY: M.E. Sharps.

Walker, H.M., Schwarz, I.E., Nippold, M.A., Irvin, L.K., & Noell, J.W. (1994). Social skills in school-age children and youth: Issues and best practices in assessment and intervention. *Topics in Language Disorders*, *14*, 70–82.

Wehman, P., Kregel, J., Sherron, P., Nguyen, S., Kreutzer, J., Fry, R., & Zasler, N. (1993). Critical factors associated with the successful supported employment of patients with severe traumatic brain injury. *Brain Injury*, *7*, 31–44.

Wehman, P.H., West, M.D., Kregel, J., Sherron, P., & Kreutzer, J.S. (1995). Return to work for persons with severe traumatic brain injury: A data-based approach to program development. *Journal of Head Trauma Rehabilitation*, *10*, 27–39.

Welsh, M.C., Pennington, B.F., & Groisser, D.B. (1991). A normative-developmental study of executive function: A window on prefrontal function in children. *Developmental Neuropsychology*, *7* (2), 131–149.

Wiener, J., & Harris, P.J. (1998). Evaluation of an individualized, context-based social skills training program for children with learning disabilities. *Learning Disabilities Research and Practice, 12,* 40–53.

World Health Organization. (1980). *International classification of impairments, diseases, and handicaps: A manual of classificaion relating to the consequences of disease.* Geneva, Switzerland: Author.

Ylvisaker, M. (1992). Communication outcome following traumatic brain injury. *Seminars in Speech and Language, 13,* 239–251.

Ylvisaker, M. (1993). Communication outcome in children and adolescents with traumatic brain injury. *Neuropsychological Rehabilitation, 3,* 367–387.

Ylvisaker, M., & Feeney, T. (1996). Executive functions: Supported cognition and self-advocacy after traumatic brain injury. *Seminars in Speech and Language, 17,* 217–232.

Ylvisaker, M., & Feeney, T. (1998a). *Collaborative brain injury intervention: Positive everyday routines.* San Diego, CA: Singular Publishing Group.

Ylvisaker, M., & Feeney, T. (1998b). Everyday people as supports: Developing competencies through collaboration. In M. Ylvisaker (Ed.), *Traumatic brain injury rehabilitation: Children and adolescents* (Rev. ed.), (pp. 429–464). Boston: Butterworth-Heinemann.

Ylvisaker, M., & Gioia, G. (1998). Cognitive assessment. In M. Ylvisaker (Ed.), *Rehabilitation following traumatic brain injury in children and adolescents* (pp. 159–179). Newton, MA: Butterworth-Heinemann.

Ylvisaker, M., Szekeres, S.F., & Feeney, T. (1998). Cognitive rehabilitation: Executive functions. In M. Ylvisaker (Ed.), *Traumatic brain injury rehabilitation: Children and adolescents* (Rev. ed.), (pp. 221–269). Boston: Butterworth-Heinemann.

Ylvisaker, M., Szekeres, S., & Haarbauer-Krupa, J. (1998). Cognitive rehabilitation: Organization and memory. In M. Ylvisaker (Ed.), *Rehabilitation following traumatic brain injury in children and adolescents* (pp. 181–220). Newton, MA: Butterworth-Heinemann.

SUGGESTED READINGS

Glang, A., Singer, G., & Todis, B. (Eds.). (1997). *Children with acquired brain injury: The school's response.* Baltimore: Paul H. Brookes Publishing.

Lyon, G., & Krasnegor, N. (1996). *Attention, memory, and executive functions.* Baltimore: Paul H. Brookes Publishing.

Meichenbaum, D., & Biemiller, A. (1998). *Nurturing independent learners: Helping students take charge of their learning.* Cambridge, MA: Brookline Books.

Ylvisaker, M. (Ed.). (1998). *Traumatic brain injury rehabilitation: Children and adolescents* (Rev. ed.). Boston: Butterworth-Heinermann.

Ylvisaker, M., & Feeney, T. (1998). Collaborative brain injury intervervention: Positive everyday routines. San Diego: Singular.

CHAPTER 6

A Perspective on Functionality for Elderly Patients and Their Caregivers

Rosemary Lubinski

Objectives

- Understand the importance of including the perspectives of elders and their family caregivers in the design and implementation of functional communication programs.
- Understand the concept of triangularization of responsibilities in setting and achieving functional approaches for elders.
- Differentiate between goals that focus on communication skills and those that focus on communication opportunities.
- Help elderly clients and their family caregivers develop a problem-solving attitude regarding communication difficulties.
- Identify and solve problems in implementing functional approaches to communication intervention with elders and their family caregivers.

INTRODUCTION

This chapter focuses on functionality for elderly patients and their caregivers. It combines the perspectives of the academic speech-language pathologist with those of the practicing clinician to create a theoretically sound and functional approach to working effectively with older adults and their caregivers in nursing homes and home health care. It also discusses some of the problems encountered in establishing a functional approach in both settings.

DEFINITION OF FUNCTIONALITY

This discussion is based on a relatively simple definition of functionality that can be applied to a continuum of assessment and intervention with older patients and their caregivers. The results of a speech-language pathologist's professional work will be functional for elderly patients and their caregivers if (1) they understand the nature of what is being done and endorse the outcomes as desirable and reasonable; (2) they have ample opportunities to apply what was worked on in therapy during the intervening time between therapy sessions and when therapy is concluded; and (3) they begin to self-generate new ways to accomplish the goals begun in therapy. This approach to functionality can be described as laying a foundation, creating opportunities for communication, and motivating problem solving. Although discussed separately, these components are not sequential but overlap in that each is being addressed throughout therapy.

Laying a Foundation

Note that the definition of functional assessment and intervention begins by including *both* the elderly patient and caregiver. Communication assessment and therapy cannot be functional unless both older patients and their significant communication partners or caregivers are included in the process. It is rare that clinicians work with elderly isolates who have little or no daily communication with family or professional care providers. Care providers are an excellent source of information regarding the communication style of older adults, their communication needs, topics, and partners, the sources of breakdown in communication, the effectiveness of strategies, and the impact of the communication disorder on their own stress and coping abilities. Including the caregiver in the assessment/intervention process creates a triangular partnership (illustrated in Figure 6–1) that provides more opportunities for strengthening therapy effectiveness. The simplicity of this figure is deceiving in that the base of the model is the dyadic relationship between the elder and his or her communication partner symbolized by the heavy black arrow. The clinician is bonded to both the elder and communication partner but stands outside their relationship and acts as teacher, facilitator, and counselor. Removal of the clinician retains the solid base that can adopt and adapt communication-enhancing and problem-solving strategies.

Inclusion of the caregiver also underscores the fact that communication is a dyadic, shared process between two people. It demonstrates that the best way to achieve communication effectiveness is to share the responsibilities between the elderly patient and those with whom he or she

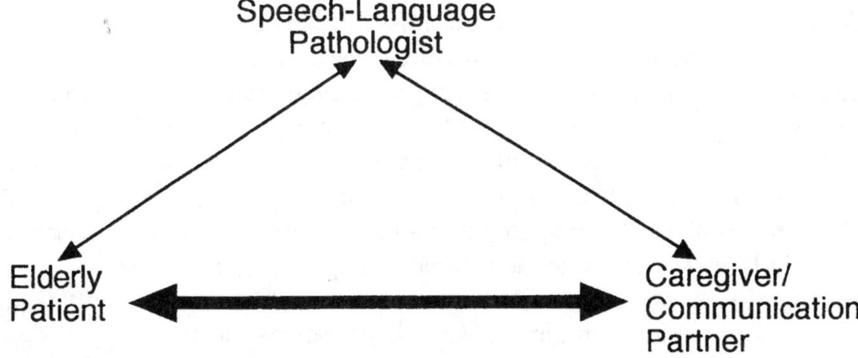

Figure 6–1 Triangularization of functional therapy.

communicates. Functionality will be achieved best when caregivers realize their own importance and responsibilities in achieving therapy goals. Finally, including caregivers in assessment and intervention gives the clinician a more realistic idea of how well elders and their caregivers understand the goals and strategies of therapy and their abilities to implement and modify strategies. It provides for more open dialogue among all parties involved.

Once the triangularization of responsibilities is established, three goals must be accomplished. The first is that the elderly patient and caregiver must understand the nature of the communication problem and provide input regarding their goals for therapy. It is the speech-language pathologist's responsibility to explain what the problem is in terminology suitable to the elder's and caregiver's educational, language, and professional background, as well as their emotional readiness to accept such information. This will lead naturally to a dialogue about the goals, methods, and expected outcomes of therapy. Such bilateral discussion not only lays a foundation for therapy but begins the transition to the problem-solving stage of functional therapy.

The current literature on functional communication assessment and intervention proposes that goals focus on the elderly patient's communication disability or handicap. It is easier for elderly patients and caregivers to understand the concept of improving communication skills, communication effectiveness, and communication opportunity. Communication skill is the ability to receive, interpret, and send messages. These skills include understanding and sending verbal and nonverbal messages, the cognitive skills necessary to formulate messages and respond, and the pragmatic skills necessary to interact competently. Effectiveness is the success a person has in receiving and sending messages irrespective of communication skill. Effectiveness involves using whatever strategies or devices are necessary to achieve interaction. Opportunity is the presence of desired partners, access to meaningful activity, and an attitude that values the participation of the person (Lubinski, 1995).

It is the clinician's job to solicit from the elderly patient and caregiver what skills are important to them, what strategies have promoted message reception and expression, and what opportunities they want to maintain or restore. The clinician might ask such questions as the following: What problems do you have in understanding what is said (read)? What problems do you have in expressing yourself through talking (writing)? What do you (patient or caregiver) do when there is difficulty in understanding or speaking? What opportunities for communication do you miss?

The answers to these questions along with the clinician's evaluation of communication will lead to a collaborative setting of goals. The clinician must then ascertain if the established intervention goals are both desirable and reasonable to accomplish. Patients, caregivers, and even clinicians may have ideal goals in mind that may be unrealistic because of such factors as the patient's level of severity, presence of complicating factors, or lack of resources to accomplish the goals. Furthermore, setting of priorities has become increasingly important in an age of managed care and limited service delivery. The clinician must quickly ascertain what skills are desired by the client and caregiver, compare these with clinician-determined goals, and create a program that incorporates the client/caregiver goals and maximizes available time and resources. Again, the active role of both elder and caregiver in this process allows for a more accurate and timely determination of priorities. It also encourages all parties to reevaluate what is possible depending on progress each week and the emergence of improved skills, more opportunities to communicate, and increasing communication adaptiveness of the elderly patient and caregiver.

Including the elder and caregiver in the decision-making process is somewhat foreign to many clients and families who expect to be given a prescription of what to do, how, and when. The approach to functional communication therapy described in this chapter does not stem from the traditional intervention model that focuses on a direct relationship between etiology and remediation or goals and methods designed exclusively by the clinician. Therapy will be more functional for the elder and caregiver when they are encouraged to participate in the decision-making process, and their ideas are included in planning a viable intervention program. In fact, the very process of asking elders and their caregivers, "What do *you* want to accomplish in speech therapy?" forces them to evaluate their needs and prioritize them. It further ingrains the idea that therapy effectiveness is a shared responsibility.

Once therapy goals are established collaboratively, the clinician has the responsibility of explaining how they might be accomplished. This is also an opportunity to reinforce the concept that all parties have responsibilities in the therapy program. As therapy methods are discussed, elders and caregivers should be encouraged to offer their own suggestions. Further, this discussion of goals and methods needs to be ongoing to further encourage elders and caregivers to reassess goals and therapy effectiveness continually.

Some may say that it would be more efficient to inform the elder and caregivers about the plan of care and proceed as rapidly as possible into the clinician-directed therapy program. Some may say that the clinician is turning over professional responsibility to the client and family. In contrast, the partnership approach is laying a foundation for a therapy program that is based on cooperation, commitment, and problem solving. It is the clinician's role to explain the nature of the communication problem, provide an accurate and realistic assessment of the client and caregiver's communication strengths and weaknesses, begin a dialogue of possible goals and therapy plans, and encourage creative thinking and commitment on the part of the elder and caregiver that will be the basis for long-term problem solving.

Creating Opportunities for Communication

It is the philosophy of many clinicians that if patients improve their communication skills, they will use these skills automatically in a variety of meaningful communication contexts. It seems plausible that increased skills will generate more communication opportunities. This view, however, does not consider several dynamic factors such as the complexity of aging, individual perceptions, and the effect of the physical and social environment. In fact, many elders reside in impoverished communication environments regardless of their ability to communicate.

It almost seems trite to say that aging is complex and affects rehabilitation. But clinicians must remember that a variety of factors affect elderly patients' communicative function and responsiveness to intervention. These include internal factors such as physical, sensory, and psychological status, and external factors such as the physical and social environment. Each elderly patient's general health, hearing and vision abilities, mobility, and dexterity will affect how the patient approaches and responds to therapy. In addition, each elderly patient will contribute his or her current mental and emotional status, which will influence ability to understand and integrate therapy suggestions. External factors such as the physical and social environment either create or hinder opportunities for meaningful communication.

The concept of a communication-impaired environment where there are few opportunities for successful, meaningful communication has been discussed elsewhere (Lubinski, 1995; Lubinski et al., 1981). Some elders have rich opportunities to communicate with partners of choice, have a variety of activities that generate stimulating and meaningful conversations, and have partners who appreciate their ideas. Unfortunately, many elders reside in long-term care settings and in the community where these communication resources are not available. Making intervention functional for these elders means that the clinician must focus not only on improving communication skills to the highest possible level, but also on enhancing the communicative environment in which the elder resides.

The philosophy of functionality for elders and their caregivers presented in this chapter is predicated upon the concept that it is inadequate to improve skills without ensuring that there will be an environment where these skills can be actualized. Some elders with communication problems have experienced communication withdrawal because they and their communication partners do not want to encounter breakdowns in interaction. It is easier to anticipate what the elder needs than be faced with a communication dilemma. It is easier to avoid interaction than problem solve how to understand or be understood. These are natural reactions, since most of us take the path of least resistance even though this path may result in loss of communicative opportunities.

Some elders have limited physical access to persons and activities that might generate conversations where they might practice their improving communication skills. These include elders who have difficulty ambulating independently, who live in settings that do not promote finding a safe way, or who are totally dependent on others for assistance. Such elders may sit in one chair for many hours each day and miss out on stimulating conversation opportunities that occur elsewhere in their environment. This situation becomes particularly problematic when significant others in the environment such as caregivers do not realize the impact of access deprivation on communication opportunities.

Some elders reside in environments where there are few partners or activities that generate the desire or need to communicate. Even when partners and activities are available, the individual may reject them for a variety of reasons including depression, language and cultural differences, prejudice, and limited adaptation to the environment. For example, the institutionalized elder may not know other residents, may perceive them as undesirable communication partners, or may have limited skills in initiating conversations with others. Further, some activities in long-term care settings actually discourage communication such as talking during a religious service, a performance, or bingo when conversation may mask the activity.

For example, a dysarthric resident of an adult care facility told the speech-language pathologist that he spoke very little each day because his roommate was severely hard of hearing, he did not like the ladies at his dining table, and his only surviving relative lived 300 miles away. He disliked most of the leisure activities available and wanted to live independently in an apartment in the community. Since this individual was fairly independent in activities of daily living, he also had limited contact with professional caregivers throughout the day. A functional approach to this individual involved addressing both his intelligibility skills and his need to find desired communication partners and activities where he could practice therapy strategies and demonstrate improvement.

Long-term care settings are not the only environments that may be communicatively impoverished. Some elders who reside in the community are truly limited in the availability of communication partners and activities. They may have few or no family members with whom to communicate on a daily basis. Some are elders whose primary caregiver is an elderly spouse who carries major responsibilities for home management and care of the patient. This individual may not perceive communication as a high priority because he or she is coping with multiple challenges of caregiving, home management, and personal difficulties.

Community-dwelling elders may not have ready and frequent access to family and friends who could serve as conversation partners. Adult children may need to divide time among their own family needs, job demands, and elderly parents. Adult children encourage the elderly patient to participate in therapy, but they do not link themselves to this process or see their participation as related to progress or carryover. Further, the cohort of friends for elderly patients may themselves have immediate, pressing needs, may relocate to other areas, or may die. Those who are nearby may visit infrequently or may feel uncomfortable when communicative breakdowns occur during interaction with the elderly, communication-impaired patient.

Nor are stimulating activities more available in the community. Remember that many community-dwelling patients have difficulty ambulating or may be dependent on others for access to activities. The primary stimulating activity in the home may be television. For elders with complicating vision or hearing problems, television may provide little stimulation. Some elders do not find television programming a source of conversation. In fact, it is not uncommon for community elders to report that they really have little to talk about with anyone. Home health care providers may be a major source of cognitive and communicative stimulation for many of these individuals.

Elders and their caregivers may not understand what the clinician means when addressing the issue of communication opportunities, topics, activities, and partners. Intervention will not be functional for these individuals unless they understand that communication skills need a communication environment in which to flourish. During each therapy session, the clinician can ask the patient and his or her caregiver how they plan to use the skills or strategies after the clinician leaves. It is helpful to pose such questions as "What activities are you going to do today?" and "Where can you use the skills we worked on?" If the answer is "none" or "I do not know," it is unlikely that what was done in therapy will be implemented either that day or when therapy is ended. With limited practice between therapy sessions, there will be less progress and fewer opportunities for self-evaluation and problem solving.

Thus, clinicians should identify what activities and partners are available to the patient and include these as part of each therapy session whenever possible. This may be done by including the caregiver in the session, role playing, or conducting the therapy session during the activities as they occur. This is an especially good opportunity for the clinician to model strategies for preventing or repairing communicative breakdowns.

Encouraging therapy in real-life contexts also helps the clinician appraise patient and caregiver understanding of the strategies and encourage creativity on their part. The clinician will then be able to fine-tune strategies and reinforce the patient and caregiver's attempts to use and adapt the strategies. The following case highlights the importance of including the caregiver in the therapy process.

> As the speech-language pathologist was about to end a period of therapy with an elderly patient with moderate Broca's aphasia, the patient's sister with whom he resided said, "That's OK, we communicate just fine. I do just what you do." This led the clinician to say "What is it that I do?" The sister, while eavesdropping from the kitchen as they did therapy in the dining room, had analyzed the strategies the clinician used to promote expression and implemented them in conversations with her brother. The clinician asked her to demonstrate them and found that the woman had chosen to pose closure-type questions to her brother that resulted in his intelligible responses. The clinician opted to extend therapy for several more sessions to focus on refining the sister's skills to prevent or repair communication difficulties with her brother.

Instilling a Problem-Solving Attitude

Therapy truly becomes functional for patients and their caregivers when they can actively assume a problem-solving attitude toward preventing or repairing communication breakdowns. For most elderly patients, therapy is not about restoring lost communication abilities to premorbid levels. It is about learning how to communicate as effectively as possible in as many desired contexts as possible. This is a shared responsibility between patients and their caregivers, with the clinician serving as facilitator or catalyst.

Thus, the speech-language pathologist's most important role is to develop in elderly patients and their caregivers a dynamic problem-solving attitude. It begins during the first encounters with the patient and caregivers, usually in an assessment context when the clinician asks such questions as: "What concerns you about your communication?" "What do you want to achieve in therapy?" "What strategies have you tried that help facilitate communication?" "What strategies work best and why?" Asking such questions gives the impression that the clinician values the patient's and caregiver's ideas and perceptions about communication. It also lays the foundation for shared responsibility and problem solving that are the real focus of therapy.

What does "problem solving" mean? Problem solving means that patients and their caregivers consciously think about and then act to make each communicative event successful. Communication is not something that just happens, but something that *they* can make happen. Each person needs to assume communication responsibility and use the skills he or she has to make effective communication thrive. Elders and their caregivers need to understand that the problem they are solving is how to send and receive messages successfully even though the structure of the message may not be perfect.

Each person brings certain resources and constraints to the communicative event. The speech-language pathologist's goal is to maximize their resources and minimize the constraints. For example, elderly husbands and wives have a long history of communicating as a couple. They are familiar with each other's ideas, verbal and nonverbal ways of expression, routines, and preferences. The clinician can remind them that they "know each other like a book." Thus, the wife should be encouraged to mentally "fill in the blanks" when her husband's speech is unclear or incomplete. She is also familiar with the physical and social environment that will influence communication topics and intentions. Caregivers should be encouarged to be good detectives or good guessers as to what the elderly person is trying to communicate.

Another resource these individuals might have is their ability to cope with adversity. The same problem-solving attitude they used to cope successfully with previous problems can be used during communicative encounters. The clinician can ask them to think back to some other difficult problems they had in their lives and to reflect on the strategies they used to solve those issues. People are more likely to use strategies that have worked previously than newly imposed ones. Some other resources they might use include prayer and contemplation and turning to family or professionals for counseling; physical, financial, or emotional assistance; or respite.

Although the list of resources any elderly patient and caregiver might call upon is considerable, one resource that clinicians should try to model is the ability to use humor. When patients and caregivers can laugh during communicative attempts, the interaction tends to be more successful. The clinician can model humor in each session and discuss it as a way to ease through the problem solving needed during difficult communicative breakdowns.

Elders and their caregivers also bring numerous constraints to their communicative exchanges. One of the most important of these constraints is depression on the part of either the elderly patient or the caregiver. Various studies indicate that between 5% and 65% of elders exhibit some degree of depression, with 20% being a commonly accepted rate (Blazer, 1986; Blazer,1989a; Butler, Lewis, & Sunderland, 1991). The prevalence of depression among clinical groups such as stroke survivors may be as high as 60% (Robinson, Starr, & Rice, 1988). In addition, family caregivers frequently experience depression. For example, Cohen and Eisdorfer (1988) found that 55% of major caregivers residing with a relative with dementia experienced clinical depression. Thus, both elders and their caregivers are at high risk for developing some degree of depression.

Depression is a rather insidious problem in that people may not recognize it, acknowledge it, or seek help for it. It can also seriously disrupt therapy participation and progress. The willingness of the patient or caregiver to assume responsibility in therapy or adopt a problem-solving attitude may be compromised. Speech-language pathologists need to be aware of the possible symptoms of depression and know how and when to refer the patient or caregiver for help. This problem must be addressed first by the patient's medical doctor if therapy is to be effective and functional. Clinical management may include removal or control of potential etiologic agents, pharmacotherapy, psychotherapy, and electroconvulsive therapy. Blazer (1989b, p. 166) states that although total recovery is not realistic for all elderly persons with depression, it is the most treatable of psychiatric disorders in later life.

Developing a problem-solving attitude on the part of the patient and caregiver begins during the first encounters with them. The clinician can explain to them that they are attacking the communication breakdowns from two perspectives. The first is enhancing the patient's communicative skills to the highest level possible and training the patient and caregiver in strategies that will promote the effective exchange of information. The second is through developing their problem-solving abilities. What is done in therapy can never duplicate exactly the variety of exchanges that will occur at other times. The patient and therapist will never practice all the words the patient may want to express; they will never duplicate in therapy the physical or psychological environment the patient will experience at other times. Thus, the patient and caregiver must know what to do when they face a communicative dilemma later in the day, tomorrow, or months from now.

Problem-solving skills can be developed by including the caregiver in therapy sessions and talking about what strategies work best for facilitating expression and comprehension. The clinician can model strategies that are transparent in their delivery, and then discuss with the patient and caregiver what strategy was used and ask them their opinion regarding its implementation and success. At this point, the clinician can solicit their suggestions for other strategies and continue to probe for their evaluation of the effectiveness of each strategy. It is also helpful to discuss what makes situations difficult and what might be done to preclude them. This problem-solving aspect of therapy overlaps nicely with continued reevaluation of goals and creation of communication opportunities outside of therapy.

WHAT THIS APPROACH DOES NOT EMPHASIZE

The approach to functional therapy described above has not delineated specific strategies for preventing or repairing conversational dilemmas. Strategies are generally specific to particular types of disorders and should be customized to meet the needs of each patient. Further, what is equally important are the strategies that the patient and the caregiver devise for themselves to maintain successful communication. The patient and caregiver need to know what they do to facilitate communication and how successful it is.

This discussion has not focused on "functional activities" such as those based on activities of daily living (for example, practice talking on the phone, conveying information about health care, etc.). It should be a given that the topics discussed and the contexts practiced will have relevance to each individual elderly patient. Therapy topics and contexts should emerge from the questions asked of the patient and caregiver and the priorities they and the clinician have set. Simply because talking on a telephone was included in an inventory of functional communication does not mean that this context is important for every patient.

This approach has also not viewed caregiver education as a separate component from working with the patient. In some therapy contexts, the clinician works individually with the patient and finds extra time to discuss progress with or "counsel" the caregiver. In the approach to functional therapy described here, the caregiver participates in an ongoing, integrated, and critical aspect of therapy. Caregiver inclusion involves education, counseling, discussions, modeling, and reinforcement. Caregivers are considered strategic partners in the therapy process and not bystanders.

PROBLEMS IN IMPLEMENTING THIS APPROACH

Many older adults approach speech-language therapy cautiously if not skeptically. They understand intuitively that what they do in physical or occupational therapy will relate to ambulation, safety, or independence in activities of daily living. Speech therapy goals and activities are not always as obvious. Further, older adults may not view improving communication as a high priority as compared to difficulties in reducing pain, walking, eating, or dressing. Elders and caregivers may be so consumed by the elder's medical or physical needs that they neglect social communicative needs. Further, they may not be accustomed to taking such an active role in determining goals, implementing strategies, planning carryover activities, or problem solving. Those who are reluctant to verbalize their goals may need help in expressing their ideas; in fact, some may say "I don't know" to many of the clinician's questions. In time and with encouragement, the vast majority of elderly patients and caregivers will feel comfortable contributing their perceptions of therapy, self-generated strategies, and progress.

This approach has emphasized including caregivers in the entire process of therapy. Some caregivers may not understand the concept of shared responsibility and feel that only the elderly patient should be included in the therapy process. Unless the caregiver accepts this responsibility, the elderly patient must assume total responsibility for improvement. Therapy will be more "functional" and more effective when therapy goals, responsibility, and problem solving are shared.

Another problem is how to incorporate caregivers into therapy on a daily basis. This is problematic when the caregiver is an adult child who lives outside the home of the patient. Spouses may feel reluctant to be a part of therapy in that their presence might be intrusive. Discussing these problems at the outset of the diagnostic and therapy program will help the clinician, patient, and caregiver decide on how and when the incorporation will be done. The clinician may need to be creative in ways to incorporate the caregiver (for example, leaving a videotape of a session with modeled strategies and commentary, or viewing a video made by the caregiver when conversing with the patient). Therapy sessions may need to be at nontraditional times that are more convenient for the caregiver.

One may also assume that this approach is only for family caregivers. It is more difficult but not impossible to implement with professional caregivers in both long-term care and home care settings. There are two ways of approaching professional caregivers—through inservice programs and through modeling communication strategies in places where caregivers are likely to hear and see what is occurring. Inservice programs that focus on lecture-type learning are not as effective in helping family or professional caregivers to understand the principles of this approach as inservice programs that emphasize discussion, demonstration, role playing, and counseling (Koury & Lubinski, 1995). Inservice training is also done each time the clinician models strategies in the presence of caregivers and discusses their utility. For example, the speech-language pathologist can conduct therapy sessions in front of the nurses' station so that staff and other residents might observe the strategies used and recognize the communication potential of the patient. In home care sessions, the clinician can invite the primary caregiver and others to sit in during part of every session—first to observe and eventually to be part of the session.

CONCLUSION

Speech-language pathologists who work with older adults face challenges. First, acute care hospitals generally offer little rehabilitation and focus primarily on assessment and stabilization of patients and preparation for speedy discharge to subacute care or to home. Speech-language pathologists have little time or opportunity to work with elderly patients or their families in this setting. Therapy at all levels of care is being scrutinized to determine if what speech-language pathologists do makes a difference in the everyday functioning of the patient and if this difference is worth the cost. Length of therapy is no longer indefinite but restricted by insurance contracts. With today's elderly population, speech-language pathologists are faced with more complicated, fragile cases and less time to accomplish goals. This will not change as the burgeoning elderly population strains our health care budgets.

The functional approach to therapy described in this chapter conforms to the constraints being placed on speech-language pathologists' service delivery. First, no approach to therapy will be successful, and certainly not functional, if the patients and primary caregivers do not understand what is happening and do not "buy in" to the goals. The approach proposed here treats the elderly patient and caregivers as real stakeholders in the therapy process. Therapy derives from the clinician's expertise *and* the aspirations of the participants.

Second, no approach to therapy will be successful, or functional, if what is done in therapy does not have direct application to the patient's everyday communication. To keep patients and caregivers committed to therapy, the strategies demonstrated and polished in therapy must result in observable success outside the therapy context. Progress must be transparent and meaningful to the parties involved, or their continued commitment will be questionable.

Finally, therapy will not be successful, or functional, if patients and caregivers cannot develop a sense of being a communication problem solver. Therapy time is limited. What the clinician, patient, and caregiver must accomplish ultimately is to create a dyad or series of dyads who know what to do when they face communication predicaments. The elderly individual and significant communication partners need to understand that therapy is not an end in itself but a means to understanding their own potential for developing problem-solving strategies.

The approach proposed in this chapter challenges speech-language pathologists to think somewhat differently about their role in therapy, how much they involve family members or significant others, and how they measure progress. This approach requires that power and decision making be shared with the elder and family. It also necessitates that the clinician understand the physical and social context in which the elderly patient resides and the impact of this context on communication opportunities. Clinicians need to match therapy activities with the real life of the patient. Clinicians need to actively and confidently assume various roles of teacher, catalyst, counselor, and environmental manipulator if therapy is to be effective and functional for current and future elders they serve.

Discussion Questions

1. Why will therapy be more functional for elders and their family caregivers if goals are jointly determined by all participants?
2. Why is developing a problem-solving attitude critical in developing functional approaches to communication intervention with elders?
3. What problems do speech-language pathologists face in developing functional approaches for elders?
4. How do speech-language pathologists measure outcomes for functional communication intervention with elders and their family caregivers?

REFERENCES

Blazer, D. (1986). The diagnosis of depression in the elderly. *Journal of the American Geriatric Society, 28*, 52–58.

Blazer, D. (1989a). Affective disorders in later life. In E.W. Busse & D.G. Blazer (Eds.), *Geriatric psychiatry*, pp. 369–401. Washington, DC: American Psychiatric Press.

Blazer, D. (1989b). Depression in the elderly. *New England Journal of Medicine, 320*, 164–166.

Butler, R., Lewis, M., & Sunderland, T. (1991). *Aging and mental health*. New York: Macmillan.

Cohen, D., & Eisdorfer, C. (1988). Depression in family members caring for a relative with Alzheimer's disease. *Journal of the American Geriatric Society, 36*, 885–889.

Koury, L., & Lubinski, R. (1995). Effective inservice training for staff working with communication impaired patients. In R. Lubinski (Ed.), *Communication and dementia*, pp. 279–291. San Diego: Singular Publishing Group.

Lubinski, R. (1995). Environmental considerations for elderly patients. In R. Lubinski (Ed.), *Communication and dementia*, pp. 257–278. San Diego: Singular Publishing Group.

Lubinski, R., Morrison, E., & Rigrodsky, S. (1981). Perception of spoken communication by elderly and chronically ill patients in an institutional setting. *Journal of Speech and Hearing Disorders, 46*, 405–412.

Robinson, R., Starr, L., & Price, T. (1984). A two year longitudinal study of post-stroke mood disorders: Prevalence and duration at six months followup. *British Journal of Psychiatry, 144*, 256–262.

SUGGESTED READINGS

Lubinski, R. (1995). *Communication and dementia*. San Diego: Singular Publishing Group.

Lubinski, R., & Higginbotham, D.J. (1997). *Communication technologies for the elderly: Vision, hearing, and speech*. San Diego: Singular Publishing Group.

CHAPTER 7

Sociocultural and Functional Perspectives on Clinical Outcomes: A Concerto for Two Pianos

Shelly S. Chabon, Dorian Lee-Wilkerson, and Noma B. Anderson

Objectives

- Describe the role of a sociocultural perspective in achieving functional outcomes.
- Demonstrate an understanding of how to research macroculture, mesoculture, and microculture and discuss their relevance to functionally based treatment.
- Identify sociocultural factors that affect developing and achieving functional outcomes for all children and discuss how the impact may vary when working with disabled children from culturally and linguistically diverse populations.
- Apply sociocultural and functional perspectives to clinical practice when interpreting data for assessment and diagnosis.
- Apply sociocultural constructs to treatment planning in order to achieve functional outcomes.

INTRODUCTION (PRELUDE)

Many readers have heard the joke about the man recovering from a terrible accident who asks his doctor if he will be able to play the piano. When the doctor assures him that once healed this should be no problem, the man responds with, "That's funny, because I couldn't play before the accident." This story reflects, in part, the focus of this chapter. That is, treatment outcomes cannot be based on unfounded assumptions about a client's interests, knowledge, or skills or—for that matter—on the clinician's own experiences and intuitions. Rather, to be functional, treatment decisions must be individually prescribed, culturally justified, and supported by evidence from appropriate research and literature. Said yet another way, the relative value of treatment for any client cannot be determined independent of the environment in which, and the audience with whom, the client functions in his or her everyday activities.

This chapter discusses clinical practice issues from a sociocultural and functional perspective and offers a model that illustrates the interconnectedness and importance of both of these constructs in speech-language pathologists' work with children who have communication problems. The profession's present interest in functional outcomes can best be realized through a corresponding emphasis on cultural knowledge.

THEME

Functionality, by definition, is clinical practice that results in language outcomes that support (1) social acceptance, (2) formal and informal learning, and (3) vocational goals (Nelson, 1998). The definition of functional language will vary, however, as the context of language use varies. What is functional language in the classroom may not be very functional on the job. Functionality is a framework useful for examining the communicative demands of social, educational, and vocational settings and for understanding the child's communicative abilities and disabilities. Questions derived from the functionality framework include the following:

- What language skills are needed for this setting?
- What purposes will these language skills serve?
- What specific impacts will the language skills have on performance in untargeted settings? (Kreb & Wolf, 1997)

Cultural consciousness is an awareness of and respect for cultural diversity. Culturally conscious perspectives make use of family and community-based values, traditions, customs, and resources to plan, implement, and evaluate treatment outcomes (U.S. Department of Education, 1994). The inclusion of cultural consciousness in the functionality framework provides the scaffold for posing questions that address culturally based issues. Such questions may include the following:

- What are the audience characteristics and how are these characteristics interpreted by a client in light of his/her sociocultural background?
- Is there audience-client congruity? If not, can it be achieved by increasing the client's knowledge about differing communication styles?
- What are the appropriate topics of talk and which aspects of language should be targeted in light of the client's sociocultural background?

Culturally conscious perspectives move intervention beyond the individual client to include broad audiences, such as the client's family, peers, teachers, employers, and strangers. Functionality makes use of these broad audiences and multiple environments to establish the relevance of clinical objectives and activities for the client, linking mastery with improvements in daily activities such as homework, grades, job success, and social competence (Kreb & Wolf, 1997). It seems clear that cultural relevance is a key characteristic of functional outcomes. That is, functionality cannot be separated from the cognitive, linguistic, and social behaviors from which it is derived or from the culture in which these behaviors occur.

First Movement: A Sociocultural Perspective on Functionality in Clinical Practice

Our schools, as well as our nation, are becoming increasingly multicultural, multiracial, and multilingual. If current trends continue, it is predicted that by the year 2020 almost half of school-age youths will be students of color (Banks & Banks, 1997). These demographic shifts underscore the need for speech-language pathologists to become sensitive to and knowledgeable about children with disabilities from culturally and linguistically diverse backgrounds. Sociocultural competence means being knowledgeable about one's own culture and the cultures of those individuals to whom one provides clinical services; the linguistic systems of one's own language and the languages of those individuals to whom one provides clinical services; and nonbiased assessment and intervention procedures that take into account the culture, language, lifestyles, and values of the client and the family. Sociocultural competence also involves respecting clients and families and working with these individuals so that they are comfortable in the service-delivery setting.

Individual clients, their families, their clinicians, and the therapeutic climate in which treatment is provided represent more than independent influences on treatment outcomes. They are all part of an integrated and complex process. Researchers and clinicians have tended to focus on either the individual or the environment. However, clinical practice is in a sense a sociocultural practice or, as Taylor (unpublished manuscript) asserts, a *sociocultural occasion*. This conviction is based on the recognition that everything that occurs in clinical practice relates to culture—beginning with the telephone inquiry for information or scheduling and continuing through the case history interview, the assessment process, the diagnosis, the setting of long- and short-term goals and objectives, the implementation of intervention approaches, and the establishment of exit criteria.

In accordance with this view, the speech-language pathologist conducts clinical tasks based upon culturally determined assumptions. The client's participation and interaction in the clinical process are also based upon culturally determined practices. The cultural contexts that have established these views about communication for the speech-language pathologist are the speech-language pathologist's own community as well as the cultural premises upon which the speech-language pathologist's assessment instruments and intervention methods and procedures (or cultural tools) have been based. There has been a tendency to assume that this cultural perspective is the only correct or sensible one. However, the client also has certain values, expectations, and assumptions related to treatment procedures and goals. Reflecting on the potential risk of cultural conflicts inherent in the intervention process, Crago (1992) poses the following question: "Are clinicians and educators caught in webs into which they themselves were socialized without understanding or interpreting what they transmit to the families that they serve?" (p. 8).

Lynch and Hanson (1992) also recognize the ways in which a professional's cultural views and values can influence his or her opinions of and manners of interacting with clients and families. They write:

> Interventionists who are members of the Anglo-European American culture, or are strongly influenced by it, may want to examine these values to determine their degree of identification with each and the extent to which these values affect their practice. For

> example, interventionists who value punctuality and careful scheduling may need to examine their frustration with families who place less emphasis on clock and calendar time. . . . Interventionists who value frugality may have trouble understanding why a family with very limited resources has just purchased a VCR. Interventionists who pride themselves in sensitive but direct communications may have difficulty with families who do not look them in the eye or those who nod "yes" when the answer is "no"; those who value privacy may have difficulty understanding why a preschooler is still sleeping in the parents' bedroom.
>
> Likewise, interventionists who do not come from the mainstream culture of the United States and are not highly identified with it must examine their values and beliefs in relation to the families that they serve. Cultures that value interdependence over independence, cooperation above competition, authority rather than permissive child rearing, and interaction more than efficiency may need to examine how these values affect their practice. For example, families who are striving to toilet train their child at a very young age, are encouraging self-feeding, and are leaving the child with nonfamily babysitters from infancy on may be puzzling to interventionists who place a higher value on interdependence than independence. Or, when a young child talks back or interrupts adult conversations, many Anglo-European American parents view the child's behavior as his or her right to personal expression. Native American, Asian, Latino and African American parents and interventionists may see the same behavior as disrespectful and obnoxious. (pp. 38–39)

Without a conscious "cultural orientation," client behaviors that differ from the clinician's normative expectations can be misinterpreted as deviant and treated punitively.

Banks and Banks (1997) assert that every person and group is both cultural and multicultural: "From the nuclear family, through early and later schooling, through peer networks, and through life at work, we encounter, learn, and to some extent help create differing microcultures and subcultures. Just as everyone learns differing variants and styles of the various languages we speak so that everybody is multilingual (even those of us who only speak English), so everybody is multicultural" (p. 34). From a sociocultural perspective, all individuals, including the client and the clinician, are members of at least three sociocultural systems: the macroculture, the mesoculture, and the microculture. The *macroculture* represents cultural background, which is the basis for many of the client's traditions, values, group experiences, group strivings, and cultural ideologies. Information that can be learned from an understanding of the macroculture includes: (1) structural and sociolinguistic rules of communication, (2) the linguistic and sociolinguistic rules for interpersonal interactions, and (3) the prevailing belief systems within the culture (such as values, ceremonies, views about health and disability). These types of insights are needed in order to infuse functionality throughout the intervention process. The *mesoculture* includes the individual's community, school, church, work, social interactions, etc. The *microculture* includes the family, both nuclear and extended, and close friends. A number of variables make up each individual's culture such as ethnicity, socioeconomic level, age, occupation, education, geography, gender, religion, race, language, disability, and talent. The degree to which these cultural variables characterize an individual and his or her family is an important consideration in treatment. Analysis of the macro-, meso-, and microcultural environments gives the speech-language pathologist a more thorough awareness of the client's communication demands and expectations than the conventional monocultural perspective.

The speech-language pathologist's role is to understand the client and family in relationship to their environments or cultures. The dynamics that exist within and among each individual client's macro-, meso-, and microcultures define the uniqueness of each client and family. Clients' individuality comes from the interplay within and among these three cultural spheres. No two clients have exactly the same views, values, beliefs, practices, expectations, and traditions since the manner in which each client functions within his or her cultural systems differs. It is, therefore, extremely important that the speech-language pathologist never stereotype or generalize about clients and that he or she attempt to appreciate each client and family as unique and to study the client's cultural systems. Such efforts will result in the speech-language pathologist gaining important insight into the client's environments and ultimately in the creation of a functional intervention plan.

The first step in understanding the values, beliefs, practices, and assumptions of other cultures is to become aware of these same dimensions in one's own macro-, meso-, and microcultures. Examples of this type of self-examination include understanding one's ethnic origins; reasons for one's family's immigration to this country; expectations and experiences upon arriving and since living in this country; values, practices, and communication styles that are influenced by one's family's culture; and the economic, occupational, and educational experiences of one's family across the generations of family members who have lived and are living in this country.

The speech-language pathologist's sociocultural frame of reference is his or her culture. Therefore, an understanding that one's own views, values, and assumptions are not universally held but are reflections of one's own cultures is essential to accepting cultural diversity. For example, once the speech-language pathologist understands that his or her views on child rearing or on the manner in which a child communicates with an unfamiliar adult are culturally determined, he or she can embrace diversity in perspectives, practices, and behaviors. A strong cognitive imperative of cultural diversity is the understanding that one's own culture's perspectives and behaviors are neither superior to, nor the standards or norms for, other cultures' perspectives and behaviors.

As the speech-language pathologist begins to learn about his or her own cultures, he or she is ready to explore the cultures of the families with whom he or she works. Steps involved in becoming culturally knowledgeable include being open-minded, wanting to learn, respecting and appreciating the concept of cultural diversity, reading and studying interactions with people from different cultures, learning the language of another culture, and participating in significant events within other cultures. Such cultural discoveries broaden speech-language pathologists' professional abilities and skills, and enrich them as individuals as well.

To study the client's and family's mesoculture, the speech-language pathologist must learn about the client's community. The speech-language pathologist may gain a better understanding of the client's community by reading the community newspaper for information about political, religious, and social issues; attending community festivals for information about local customs, informal interaction styles of adults and children in the community, food preparation and consumption, styles of dress, and forms and styles of communication. The speech-language pathologist may also attend PTA or parent support groups to network with parents and significant others in the community. The experiences are especially clear if the client lives in a community that is culturally different from the one where the speech-language pathologist resides. One important variable in the mesoculture is that of cultural density—whether there is a critical cultural mass. A client and family from a culture different from the U.S. cultural and linguistic mainstream, living in a community where there are only a few or perhaps no other families from a similar cultural and linguistic background, may exist within a different mesocultural system than a family living in a community where many families from similar cultural and linguistic backgrounds reside. Some excellent resources for guiding the speech-language pathologist in reviewing cultural and ethnic macroculture and mesoculture include *Developing Cross-Cultural Competence* by Lynch and Hanson (1992); *Developing Culturally Competent Programs for Children with Special Needs* (Roberts, 1990); and Saville-Troike's (1978) compilation of questions for gaining an in-depth understanding of cultural factors, family, and community (see Appendix 7–A). Answers to the questions in Saville-Troike's listing will provide a link to incorporating functionality in assessment and intervention.

Examination of the client's microculture and the communication expectations of this microculture will provide the speech-language pathologist with the data needed to develop appropriate functional goals and outcomes that will be meaningful for the client and the family. Taylor, Payne, and Anderson (1987) have presented a sample listing of the types of preassessment questions that can be considered. According to these authors, questions that can be asked of parents and caregivers include the following:

- Who is in your family?
- Who interacts most often with your child?
- Describe how your child talks and responds to adults.
- Describe how long it takes for your child to begin to engage in conversation with an unfamiliar person (i.e., length of warm-up time).
- How does your child express his/her wants and needs?
- How does your child express his/her likes and dislikes?
- How does your child begin and end conversations?
- Who tells stories to the child?
- What kinds of narratives are told and read to your child? Stories? Fairy tales? Folk tales?
- How does your child ask for information?
- What conversational topics are appropriate and which are inappropriate for your child?
- What are the styles of communication within your home?

Taylor, Payne, and Anderson (1987) suggest that observations about culture and communication for the speech-language pathologist to explore include the following:

- What are the communication style(s) of individuals when they are communicating with others from their cultural group?
- What are the conversational style(s) of individuals when communicating with others from the dominant culture as well as from other cultures?
- Is silence used as a communicative device? If so, in what ways?
- How are narratives structured? Are they topic centered or topic associative or circular? Are proverbs used in the community?
- How are conversations structured? What are the rules of turn-taking?

These questions and observations explicitly relate language to content, to environments, and to culture.

Familiarity with the client's environments is a function of the speech-language pathologist being a responsible communication ethnographer. Battle (1997) provides guidelines for ethnographic assessment with culturally and linguistically diverse clients. Ethnographic assessment enables the speech-language pathologist to examine the client's microculture. It can assist in expanding the speech-language pathologist's understanding of and appreciation for the community norms, values, and operating practices that influence the production and interpretation of speech and language (Bauman and Sherzer, 1989).

Battle's guidelines (1997) assist the speech-language pathologist in exploring the influence of culture and environment upon the child's development of language in the home and in exploring the communication behaviors important to the family. They include the following: (1) observe the child over time in multiple contexts with multiple communication partners; (2) interview members of the family network to collect data regarding the child's language skills in the home environment; (3) interact with the child, being sensitive to his or her need to create meaning based on his other frame of reference and life experiences; (4) describe the client's use of language during genuine communication in a naturalistic environment with low anxiety and high motivation; (5) describe the child's use of language in both high contextualized and low contextualized material; and (6) collect narrative samples using wordless books, pictures, and other materials (1997, p. 400).

Second Movement: A Functional Perspective on Sociocultural Diversity in Clinical Practice

Functionality is embedded in the context of social relationships and clinical practices. Participation in culturally valued activities is essential for achieving skill, understanding, and insight about treatment goals. Functional outcomes are neither "isolated" nor "universal," but rather reflect individual achievements that involve emotions and social interactions within a cultural context.

Individual or personal client variables that may moderate the effects of treatment are numerous and include self-motivation; interest; self-image; physical capabilities and disabilities; age; primary disorder; social status; and cultural, linguistic, and educational background (Cornett & Chabon, 1988). Therapist characteristics that may be determinants of successful outcome include skill, knowledge, theoretical orientation, objectivity, security, honesty, commitment to the client, patience, creativity, and cultural/linguistic background and sensitivity (Parloff, Waskow & Wolfe, 1978). Any or all of these factors may influence each other as well as the relationship between the client and clinician, which ultimately is a possible determinant of successful treatment outcome.

Much of the research on treatment effectiveness and functional outcomes has examined only what occurs during the actual treatment session. However, events occur outside of treatment that may have a positive or negative impact on the client and that can interact with the therapy process. Examples of such external or environmental factors include activities in which the client engages outside of the therapy hour and how he or she relates treatment to these activities; the presence or absence of a supportive network; the attitudes and involvement of significant others in the change process; and events such as academic or vocational successes or failures, a job change, a relocation, or the birth or death of a loved one. In addition, speech-language pathologists must consider the client's experiences with racism and prejudice. From this discussion, it should be clear that cultural and linguistic backgrounds are integral to, and reflective of, client variables, clinician variables, the therapeutic relationship, and variables external to the treatment session; thus, they may have a profound impact on treatment outcomes. In this view, functionality is defined as individualistic and yet is apparent only within a broader cultural, historical, and institutional framework.

Clinical activities are based upon goals and desired outcomes. Their meaning and purpose must be understood by, and compatible with, the will of the individual client and relevant to the client's cultures in order to achieve functionality. The concept of sociocultural authenticity (Damico, Smith, & Augustine, 1996) is important in directing speech-language pathologists to develop functional goals because it involves the use of "real language for real purposes in real situations" (Damico & Hamayan, 1992).

Authenticity focuses on linguistic realism, ecological validity, and representativeness (Damico, Smith, & Augustine, 1996). The term *linguistic realism* refers to the use of the client's actual utterances or "language in context" in assessment and intervention procedures. This requires knowledge of the linguistic features of the client's communication system. Among other things, such an approach enables the speech-language pathologist to explicate culture-specific communication style differences that may be misunderstood by teachers and other health care professionals, thereby enhancing the interaction between communication and academic and/or vocational performance.

The second aspect of authenticity, *ecological validity*, refers to the necessity to embed assessment and intervention processes into the client's everyday activities and naturalistic settings (Damico, Smith, & Augustine, 1996). Romski and Sevcik (1996) acknowledge that assessment of the client's environments is essential to evaluating and planning for functionality in the communication intervention process. Specifically, these authors have identified six steps for assessing the client's communication environments

1. Identify the familiar and unfamiliar partners for communication in each of the child's environments.
2. Describe the opportunities, by frequency and type, for communication typically observed in each of the child's environments.
3. Compare the opportunities for communication among the different environments and partners within each environment.
4. Determine the proportion of communications that are appropriate and inappropriate in each environment.
5. Identify specific communicative content, forms, and functions that might be useful in each environment.
6. Identify the partners in each environment who have relatively high rates of positive and interactive communications with the child.

Ecological assessments such as the one outlined by Romski and Sevcik must be conducted in naturalistic environments, and the end products are individualized functional goals and objectives (McCormick, 1997). Ecological assessment is based upon the recognition that individuals cannot be studied apart from their environments (McCormick, 1997). Two basic assumptions of the ecological assessment model are: (1) every individual is an inseparable part of a social system, and (2) a disability is a discrepancy between the individual's abilities and the expectations or demands of the environments. Ecological validity underscores the importance of selecting contexts and behaviors that are representative of the client's environments. It provides the clinician with the opportunity to make instructional materials and treatment outcomes more relevant to the needs of diverse students.

Representativeness, the final aspect of authenticity (Damico, Smith, & Augustine, 1996), refers to the need to ensure that behaviors observed in assessment and targeted for change are valid indicators of the client's actual ability. An appropriate question to ask about the representativeness of a client's performance might be: Is this client one who can't or who won't comply with a given request? The answer to this query can best be determined through the use of representative samples of behavior and only when the clinician distinguishes among behaviors that reflect a client's best, worst, or most typical performances (Damico, Smith, & Augustine, 1996; Nelson, 1998; Silliman & Wilkinson, 1991, 1994). Analysis of performance across this behavioral range enables the clinician to plan for and build on learning and communication differences in styles that may affect the rate and amount of behavioral change.

A functional approach permits the speech-language pathologist to establish priorities for improvement of communication skills. Determining where to begin in treatment and establishing end points can be difficult, if not impossible, unless there are identifiable outcomes that help pinpoint those behaviors most likely to create a desired and positive impact on a client's everyday functioning.

To be functional, clinical work should be evidence-based—that is, supported by observations made in previous successful practices as well as normative population data. Accordingly, clinical activities can be justified and clinical outcomes may be predicted (Kreb & Wolf, 1997). One of the limitations of evidence-based practice is that there often is not enough evidence to predict successful outcomes with all cultural groups. Unlike physiological responses to stimuli that undergird the use of evidence-based practice in medicine, language and communication responses to social and behavioral stimuli are much less predictable. Further, while evidence-based practice provides a systematic manner for developing treatment goals and is a useful tool for planning functional language outcomes, its value is sharply reduced without consideration of cultural differences in performance.

The plan for using evidence-based practice to establish functional outcomes usually involves measuring functional end points in terms of intermediate outcomes, instrumental outcomes, and ultimate outcomes. According to Kreb and Wolf (1997), *intermediate outcomes* are behaviors that are mastered in individual sessions such as the ability to produce three-word utterances. *Instrumental outcomes* are behaviors that signal independent use of skill. Instrumental outcomes include the ability to paraphrase passages to demonstrate comprehension, the ability to request clarification when needed, or the ability to identify syntactical errors when proofing written assignments. *Ultimate outcomes* are functionally and culturally determined and demonstrate the impact of the newly acquired skill upon activities of daily living. For example, an ultimate outcome may be that the client effectively and efficiently uses the APPLE TALK Communicator (manufactured by Prentice Romich Company, Wooster, Ohio) to express mealtime needs without assistance.

Roberts and Hutchison (1998), based on the work of Audrey Holland, suggest the addition of the phrase "in order to" to convert a clinical goal into a functional goal, because these words reflect on how an objective will affect actual performance. An example of a functional goal that incorporates such terminology is "The client will improve speech discrimination skills *in order to* understand unfamiliar speakers" (Roberts & Hutchison, 1998). Thus, the creation of functional, culturally relevant goals that promote authenticity in speech-language intervention make speech-language pathologists accountable for their client's real-life changes.

The Theme Visualized

Both the sociocultural and functional perspectives are necessary for the creation of functional clinical models. Figure 7–1 illustrates the interconnectedness of these perspectives. Functional outcomes must be developed from clinical practice that is socioculturally sound, and the functional outcomes that come from clinical practice must themselves be

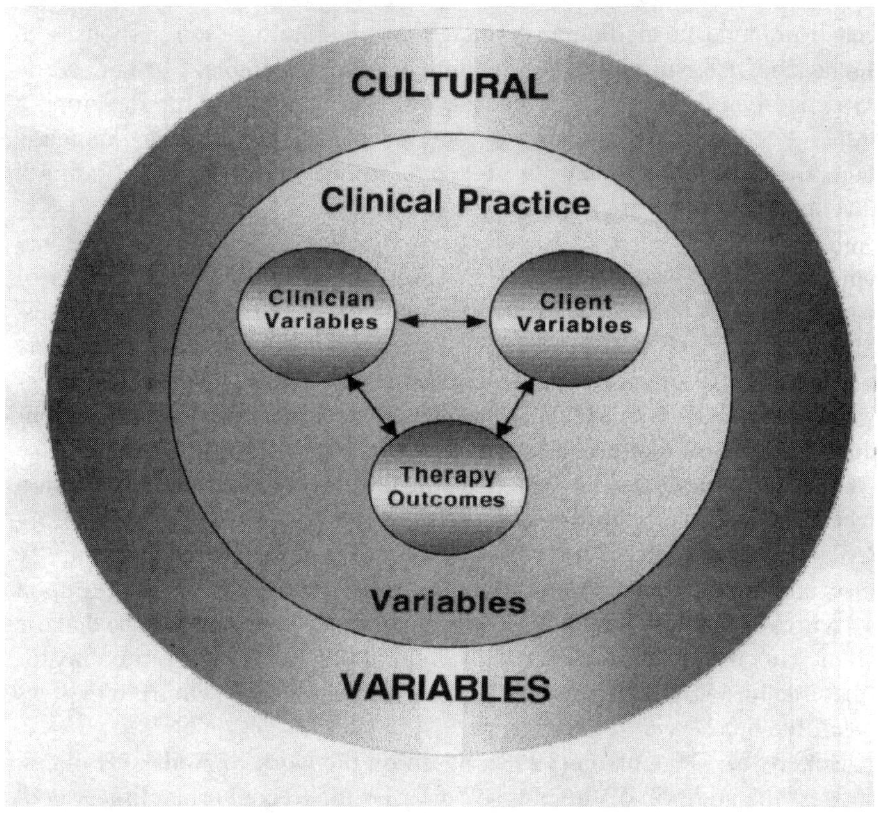

Figure 7–1 A sociocultural functionality framework.

socioculturally sound. This premise is based on the following understanding: (1) the client and family, as well as the clinician, come to the clinical setting with individual values and assumptions that are culturally based; and (2) the client and family, as well as the clinician, have macro-, meso-, and microcultural backgrounds that define their individual uniqueness. The clinician, a product of his or her cultural environments, brings to the clinical process a theoretical orientation reflective of academic preparation and knowledge base; clinical methods and materials from the clinician's professional experiences; and his or her personal qualities (such as creativity, sensitivity, objectivity, honesty, commitment, and patience). The client, a product of his or her cultural environments, comes to clinical practice with another, perhaps different cluster of variables. Each client's uniqueness determines to a great extent his or her expectations about intervention, motivation, value placed upon assessment and intervention, the effort expended (for example, a family of three young children who with their mother take two buses and a subway train each way so one of the children can attend a 50-minute therapy session twice a week), and the degree of comfort and trust felt.

Although cultural values, beliefs, and practices significantly influence functional outcomes, they may be considered less routinely by clinicians. Most speech-language pathologists are aware that culture colors intervention and influences treatment outcomes. Yet, all too often, consideration of cultural influences upon treatment outcomes is an afterthought. Moreover, many clinicians believe that once a functional intervention method has been adopted, pertinent cultural issues will be addressed automatically. In contrast, a socioculturally competent clinician is one who is actively aware of the client's sociocultural environments and the client's orientation to the clinical setting. Correspondingly, a socioculturally competent clinician is consciously aware of his or her own sociocultural environments and his or her own professional and personal orientations to the clinical setting.

FOUR PART INVENTION

The following four case studies illustrate the need for interventionists to address cultural issues together with functional issues in planning for functional clinical outcomes. In each example, the results of intervention were improved by incorporating both perspectives.

Case 1: Treatment Outcomes Reflect Multiple Cultural/Linguistic Environmental Contexts

The first case involves a 12-year-old male student who lived with his maternal aunt and uncle and three cousins. The case history is sketchy; according to caregiver report and school records, the child was doing well in school and at home until the fifth grade. Early in the school year, the child was repeatedly tardy or absent. When in class, he was often noncompliant and verbally aggressive. This seemingly sudden change in behavior prompted the request for a complete assessment. The child was tested at age 10 years, 6 months. The results of the psychological and educational evaluations were inconclusive, because the child was uncooperative during the testing procedures. The social evaluation revealed that the child had attended three different elementary schools in six years due to family relocations. No other information was available. The results of the speech and language evaluation were also inconclusive. The only formal test completed was the *Peabody Picture Vocabulary Test, Form III* (Dunn & Dunn, 1997). Results indicated that the student exhibited a two-year delay in receptive vocabulary acquisition.

Although the child was observed to be truant, noncompliant, and aggressive, he was willing to work with the speech-language pathologist in an individual setting, and was placed on her caseload. Additional baseline testing noted weaknesses in comprehension of complex semantic relations, limited syntactic knowledge, and failure to attend to structured tasks. The recommended goals were as follows:

- to define kindergarten through fourth-grade-level words—80% of trials
- to produce oral and written sentences—80% of trials—and to produce oral and written stories of 10 or more sentences

The expected *instrumental* goals were:

- to use word knowledge to comprehend oral directions in class—80% of lessons assigned
- to produce grammatically correct sentences in written assignments—80% of trials
- to produce expository narratives for language arts and history assignments—80% of trials.

The expected *ultimate* goals included:

- increased completion of in-class and homework assignments
- improved academic performance

The speech-language pathologist elected to use narratives as the method of instruction for several reasons. First, this child had lost interest in school, so stories were used to gain his attention and to provide a forum for discussion of his concerns in the context of increasing semantic and syntactic skills. Second, oral and written narratives were used to facilitate the targeting of syntactic rules in a nonthreatening manner. Syntactic rules (such as subject-verb agreement and clause formation) were illustrated by emphasizing story grammar (Pelligrini, Galda, & Rubin, 1984). Third, the use of narratives facilitated active participation of the student in the treatment process. Rather than teaching syntactic and semantic rules, the child was taught strategies to analyze narratives in order to discover the syntactic rules applied and the meanings expressed.

Therapy was implemented over a 12-week period. The sessions were 30 minutes of individual treatment, twice a week. Oral narratives were presented, and written narratives were also read to the student. At times, the student read along with the clinician. Topics were selected from history, geography, and language arts units from the school's curriculum. Themes included biographies of historical figures and current personalities, current events, cultural celebrations, and world geography.

Vocabulary was targeted using a modified version of the Word Identification Strategy (Lenz, Schumaker, Deshler, & Beals, 1984). For oral stories, new vocabulary was introduced by spelling a word, identifying its morphological structure, defining it, and giving examples of its use in sentences. For written stories, the student and clinician perused the text to identify the vocabulary targets, to identify the morphological structure, and to discover meaning via its use in the story sentences. After reading or listening to each story, the student was asked to describe in his own words the meaning of the targeted vocabulary words as they were used in the story.

The story grammar was analyzed by identifying examples of subject-verb agreement and use of clauses with conjunctions. The student practiced formulation of oral and written sentences using subject and verb, in accordance with Standard American English, and formulation of oral and written sentences with conjunctions.

The student was also instructed to analyze the narrative structure by identifying the character and the setting, retelling the plot, and stating the conclusion with the clinician's assistance and use of a story analysis chart. Strategies were given for describing the characters and identifying the setting, plot, and conclusion.

In the final task of each session, the child was to write a narrative of four or more sentences summarizing the story or topic discussed that day. The student formulated original sentences using the vocabulary presented in any of the sessions. The components of the story analysis chart provided the student with an outline for creating the narrative.

Mastery of new vocabulary did not progress beyond 50% accuracy for words at the kindergarten through second-grade level. Production of written sentences using subject-verb agreement in Standard English reached a 70% accuracy level. Production of oral sentences reached an accuracy level of 50%. Independent story analysis was never achieved. The student resisted this activity repeatedly, and he did not attain progress beyond character identification.

This case example may represent a failure to link *academic* language with *home* language. All tasks created for intervention were academic in nature. All materials selected came from the curriculum. Even the method of story analysis was taken from the performance evaluation component of the curriculum. Although it is important to "enhance the interaction between communication and academic performance" (American Speech-Language-Hearing Association, 1997), this may not be readily accomplished if cultural factors are not considered.

During the next 12-week treatment period, a different therapeutic approach was used. This approach made use of both a cultural and a functional perspective. The clinician gathered samples of oral stories from the student's peers as well as published stories from writers representative of the student's cultural groups. The student read and/or listened to the stories and analyzed them. The clinician modified the story analysis chart to better describe the structure used in some of the stories gathered from the student's community. The modified analysis chart asked the student to specify the characters, relationships, events, the relationships between characters and events, relations between events, and the underlying theme of the story. The student read and listened to additional stories originating from the school's culture, as well. These stories were also analyzed, but using the unmodified story analysis chart. The student compared and contrasted the different narrative structures encountered using the story analysis chart.

The clinician continued to target vocabulary using the word identification strategy. New words were introduced via a variety of storytelling styles. Story grammar was targeted. The student identified the dialects used, described the grammatical rules, and made comparisons between Standard English and other varieties of English.

The student and clinician engaged in brainstorming to select themes for student-created stories from home experiences, stories read in therapy, and the school's curriculum. Student-created stories were first accomplished with the assistance of the clinician and story analysis chart, then without the assistance of the clinician. The student used photography (Tarulli, 1998) to create stimuli to add to character description and story development. He took these photographs in classrooms, in school corridors, in the cafeteria, in the gymnasium, and on the school grounds. The student created additional stories by changing the plot of stories read in different classes and by describing his unique interpretations of historical events. He was also asked to create stories based on locations studied in geography class.

Clinical Outcomes

The student now defines kindergarten through second-grade-level words in 100% of trials, and third-grade-level words in 50% of trials. The student can identify syntactic errors in oral and written sentences in 90% of trials. The student can tell stories of 10 or more sentences using the targeted grammatical structures when given pictorial stimuli and a story analysis chart.

Functional approaches assist the child with making links between therapeutic language activities and classroom activities. Some children also need bridges to help them make the link between home language and school language. Sociocultural functionality approaches help children recognize ways in which they can use knowledge gleaned from home experiences to understand and make use of the new concepts learned in school. In the case example just presented, the student may have benefited from hearing and analyzing stories from his home culture. This experience may have validated for him that he, indeed, had some knowledge of how to tell a story and how to communicate an idea. This validation may have led to increased confidence and a willingness to learn to understand different types of stories or narratives. Language intervention programs that emphasize sociocultural functionality encourage children to draw on their home experiences to support academic and language learning. They also encourage children to risk exposure to unfamiliar experiences and new ways of thinking to support academic and language learning (Knapp, Thurnball, & Shields, 1990).

Language outcomes matched with classroom learning and home learning activities are more likely to lead to improvement in academic performance. The speech-language pathologist consults with the classroom teachers, academic support personnel, parents, family, peers, and significant persons in the community. The speech-language pathologist wants to know the types of learning activities provided, the types of learning styles expected, the types of communicative styles best suited for learning in the classroom, and the anticipated learner outcomes. Additionally, the speech-language pathologist wants to know about home and community activities that include the child. Asking questions about recreational and religious activities, family roles and responsibilities, and peer group affiliations will give the speech-language pathologist information about the language and communication skills expected outside of the classroom. This information will also alert the speech-language pathologist if there is a mismatch between home and school language, communication, and learning styles. If there is a mismatch, the speech-language pathologist can plan to teach the child strategies for managing such mismatches. In doing this, the child's language outcomes are more likely to be functional in multiple settings.

Case 2: Treatment Outcomes Based on Cultural/Linguistic Background Information from Several Sources

The second case example illustrates what happens when the clinician does not have enough information about the client's background to facilitate therapeutic progress. It involves a 12-year-old male with a history of pre- and postnatal drug exposure. He also experienced physical abuse and neglect during infancy and early childhood. This child reportedly performed within the borderline-normal range for cognitive functioning as measured by the Wechsler Intelligence Scale for Children, Revised (Wechsler, 1974) and was described as easily distracted. On the Clinical Evaluation of Language Fundamentals—Revised (Semel, Wiig, & Secord, 1987), his performance yielded a total language score of 77, a percentile rank of 6, and a language age equivalent of 8 years, 9 months. Language strengths appeared to be knowledge of word classes, word structure, and sentence structure. Language weaknesses were following oral directions and formulating sentences. This child had knowledge of language form and content, but he failed to use it effectively—especially for academic tasks.

Two recommended intermediate goals were (1) following two- and three-step oral directions in 80% of trials and (2) following two-, three-, and four-step written directions in 80% of trials. The expected instrumental outcomes included (1) following oral and written directions for completion of in-class assignments in 80% of trials; and (2) following oral and written directions for completion of home assignments in 80% of trials.

Thirty-minute individual treatment sessions were held twice a week for 12 weeks. The treatment strategies selected were positive practice and feedback. Within six weeks, the student was able to follow three-step oral directions with 90% accuracy and four-step written directions with 80% accuracy during his individual sessions. Once this performance level was obtained, a class log was developed to track the student's ability to follow in-class directions and directions for homework assignments. The in-class log was developed to track completion of assignments in mathematics and language arts. A homework log was developed for all assignments; the student kept the data. The clinician verified the accuracy of the log with classroom teachers on a weekly basis for a period of four weeks. During the tracking period, the student completed only 50% of home assignments with assistance and 75% of class assignments within the two targeted classes with some assistance ("some assistance" was defined as gentle reminders to complete tasks).

The clinician analyzed the homework log to determine which factors were contributing to the low rate of completion of homework assignments. The analysis did not reveal any significant factors. It seemed that neither the academic subject, the type of homework assignment given, length of directions, nor the day of the week contributed to the rate of homework completion.

In case 2, factors interfered with the client's completion of homework that were unknown to the clinician. Standard interviews with the client, family, and teachers did not provide information about why the rate of completed homework assignments was low.

Some significant background information may be overlooked using traditional approaches for gathering case history. Culturally conscious approaches seek background information from varied sources. In case 2, the student's treatment was restructured using attitudinal and perceptual information to formulate goals and select treatment strategies.

The "corners" technique developed by Andrini (1991) uses a Likert-type scale to discover the attitudes and interests of students when gathering background information. With "corners," a statement is read in which the student responds by choosing "strongly agree," "agree," "disagree," or "strongly disagree." The scale is usually administered to groups of students. After administration of the scale, the students discuss and compare their responses to determine similarities and differences among themselves. In the second case example, a modified "corners" procedure was used. First, a group of students from the client's class and the client brainstormed the topic: *factors that prevent the completion of homework.* They identified several reasons for not completing homework, including after-school job responsibilities, lack of private space in the home, having to care for siblings or offspring, unclear directions, lost textbook, lack of paper and pens, forgetting the assignment, lack of interest in assignment, better things to do. The brainstorming activity was also repeated with other students in language therapy and with a group of college students. Statements from the brainstorming sessions were used to compose an attitudinal scale for the client to complete. The results of the scale revealed that several factors were interfering with his completion of homework assignments. The student failed to comprehend the language used in mathematics for problem solving and frequently forgot to take home correct textbooks. In addition, the student failed to do homework at the same time every evening. These patterns were not evident in the homework log. While the homework log proved effective for tracking the percentage of completed homework assignments, it was not effective for identifying factors that determined why the student's homework completion rate was so low. The "corners" technique proved useful in identifying such factors.

Based on analysis of the homework log and the results of the "corners" procedure, the treatment plan was changed to address the issue of following directions to complete homework assignments. Treatment goals remained the same, but treatment strategies were modified. In response to the issue of failure to comprehend math assignments, the treatment plan included strategies for increasing vocabulary, in individual 30-minute sessions. The plan targeted measurement terms, analysis relationships, and temporal relations. The student and clinician also developed a plan for managing homework. The plan involved writing on a note card which textbooks to take home each afternoon. The student placed the note card in his pocket and checked each day before leaving his locker at the end of the day. Another client, acting as a buddy, was assigned to the client. The client and the buddy had the responsibility of reminding each other to make the note card and to check it at the end of the day. The management plan also included the amount of time to spend on each assignment, a strategy for moving onto the next assignment, a reminder to check whether the previous assignment was completed, and a strategy for turning in incomplete assignments along with a list of questions to get additional help from the teacher. In addition, the student set aside a specific time in the evening for doing homework (in consultation with parents).

Progress data indicates that the student now completes 70% of homework assignments. For those assignments not completed, the student submitted what he was able to complete with a list of questions soliciting more help. Sometimes the questions were general requests for additional help. At other times, specific questions about clarity of word meaning or the correct sequence of actions to take to complete the assignment were included. Based on these requests, the student began receiving tutoring during study hall. The homework management plan also increased parental involvement, and the buddy plan increased peer cooperation. The student continues to require assistance with completing assignments, but this results more often from student-initiated requests. Increased comprehension of measurement terms was also documented. Initially, the student failed to comprehend any of the 10 measurement terms targeted. Posttreatment data yielded a performance level of 90%. The student completed analogies with 75% accuracy and comprehended sentences using temporal relations with 80% accuracy.

Case 3: Treatment Outcomes Compatible with the Client's Cultural Preferences and Language Learning Styles

This Caucasian student, 12 years of age, was diagnosed with a learning disability and conduct disorder. The Test of Language Development-Intermediate (Hammill & Newcomer, 1988) was administered. The student performed in the 50th percentile for vocabulary and grammatical comprehension, 25th percentile for generals, 16th percentile for malapropisms, and 9th percentile for word ordering. These language scores suggest that the student demonstrated average functioning in the areas of sentence comprehension and vocabulary. His performances in categorizing concepts, formulating sentences, identifying grammatical errors, and identifying phonological errors were below average. Written language samples provided little information, as this student resisted attempts to elicit written samples in individual and class settings. The samples that were elicited were limited in size, ranging from one to five sentences in length. Sentence length in conversation ranged from five to seven words, and sentence types only included simple and compound structures. This student was generally noncompliant for most tasks in class, requiring extensive prompting to elicit participation.

The student refused all individual language intervention sessions. Thus, he received language therapy for 12 weeks, one time per week, for one hour, in a group setting. The group consisted of three other male students of similar age and diagnoses who were also members of the student's language arts class. Two of the group members were African American and one was Hispanic. The speech-language pathologist teamed with the language arts teacher to target the individual language goals stated in the student's individualized educational plan. The language arts curriculum was used as a source for treatment materials. The following language goals were targeted:

- The student will produce oral narratives summarizing the main idea, ranging from 5 to 10 sentences in length in order to demonstrate comprehension of assigned reading.
- The student will produce written narratives on a topic, ranging from 5 to 10 sentences in length in order to demonstrate written communication skills.
- The student will produce complex sentences containing coordinating conjunctions in 80% of trials, in order to demonstrate effective written communication.
- The student will produce complex sentences containing subordinating conjunctions in 80% of trials, in order to demonstrate effective written communication skills.

The expected impact upon academic performance included increased class participation, increased reading comprehension, completion of in-class written assignments, and increased frequency of oral and written expression.

The treatment strategies selected were the RAP strategy (Schumaker, Deshler, & Denton, 1984), proofing of written narratives, and sentence formulation trials. In the term RAP, the "R" refers to read the paragraph, the "A" refers to ask yourself what the paragraph is about, the "P" refers to put in your own words a statement about the main idea of the paragraph along with a statement that provides two supporting details. The RAP strategy was modified to provide the student with a rationale and topics for producing oral and written narratives. According to RAP, the student reads a paragraph; asks himself, "What was the paragraph about?"; identifies the main idea; formulates a sentence to express that main idea; and formulates one or more additional sentences to express supporting details about that main idea. The sentences were used as a basis to create either expository or persuasive oral and written narratives. Syntactic goals were targeted during oral and written sentence formulation trials and during proofing exercises with the written narratives.

The clinician introduced the RAP strategy using a "think-aloud" technique, or "talking" through the implementation of the strategy. Next, the student was given a pretest consisting of reading a paragraph, identifying the main idea, and giving two supporting details. Five trials were given and scored in terms of the student's ability to identify the main idea and supporting details, to provide meaningful information, to formulate original sentences, and to formulate complex sentences (Schumaker, Deshler, & Denton, 1984). The next step involved teaching the student to use the strategy to improve his abilities to formulate oral and written narratives based on assigned readings. Teaching methods included having the student describe the strategy, direct the clinician in its use, and direct peers in its use. The student was encouraged to use the think-aloud technique when directing others. There were also practice trials using the strategy—beginning with easy-to-read, short paragraphs and advancing to lengthy, complex materials. Five paragraphs were presented at each session. The student was assisted to recognize the main idea by locating cues that signaled the topic sentences and locating cues, such as headings and key words found in bold or italicized print, that aided in interpreting the topic sentence and identifying the main idea. A posttest was given at the end of a 12-week period. The posttest was the same as the pretest in terms of length and complexity, but different stories were used.

The student continued to be somewhat noncompliant. Some progress was noted in that the student listened to others in the group read and he offered oral statements to express the main idea six times during 12 group sessions.

Case 3 exemplifies failure to establish client ownership of the treatment plan. In this case, the speech-language pathologist collaborated well with the language arts teacher to establish the language goals and treatment strategies, but did not consult with the client. There is likely to be less resistance to intervention when clients are involved in the development and implementation of the treatment plan (Deshler & Putnam, 1996).

The clinician planned the second 12 weeks of treatment by having the client's group discuss and/or list situations in which it would be useful to have the ability to produce different types of narratives, the elements that would make the narrative effective, and whether oral or written narratives would be the most appropriate. Following this planning session, new treatment goals were formulated. The new goals included the following:

- The student will produce oral narratives stating the main idea and three or four important details, ranging from 5 to 10 utterances in length in order to summarize assigned readings to help a friend complete his homework.
- The student will produce written narratives on the assigned topics, ranging from 5 to 10 sentences in length, in order to complete history home assignments.
- The student will produce complex sentences containing required conjunctions in 80% of trials, in order to produce flyers advertising after-school dance fund-raisers.
- The student will produce complex sentences containing required conjunctions in 80% of trials, in order to produce comic strips for inclusion in the monthly student newsletter.
- The student will produce oral and written narratives, ranging from one to five utterances in length in 80% of trials, in order to produce weekly school announcements over the public announcement system.
- The student will produce one written narrative, ranging from 100 to 250 words in length, per month in order to produce a monthly "Happenings in Our School" newsletter.

Case 3 also exemplifies an error of overgeneralization or stereotyping based upon partial information about a client's cultural background. The speech-language pathologist assumed that since the student was Caucasian, mainstream values and styles of communication were appropriate frames of reference for interpreting his behaviors. The speech-language pathologist assumed that this student's learning style was compatible with instructional methods that used decontextualized language and teacher-directed tasks. Although it was true that the student's macroculture and microculture were mainstream, he attended an integrated school. The school's critical cultural mass was mainstream, but the influence of African-American and Hispanic cultures was strong. Most times, professionals view the school as reflective of mainstream culture. At one level it is, but children bring to school elements of their home culture, and these elements influence the school's culture. Depending on the cultural density of the class and the cultural background of the teacher, mainstream cultural rules may or may not be operating in a particular classroom.

The student's initial response to treatment suggested that a change in treatment strategy was needed. It was noted that the student only participated in the group sessions. Based on this observation, the treatment strategy was changed to make greater use of peer-directed activities and to promote student selection of therapy materials. These strategies have been found to be effective with culturally and linguistically diverse populations (Oller, 1983).

Progress data at the end of the second 12-week session showed that the student is now willingly participating in peer-directed group sessions. He produces written complex sentences without error in 80% of trials. He uses the RAP strategy with peer assistance to summarize readings and is able to write narratives independently, one to five sentences in length. This student completes all history home assignments in study hall with peers. He can summarize orally a reading by stating the main idea and two or three important details. He works actively with peers to create the flyers, comic strips, and weekly public announcements. He has also produced one narrative for the student newsletter with peer and clinician assistance.

Case 4: Functional Outcomes Derived from an Ethnographic Assessment of Cultural/Linguistic Behaviors

A four-year-old Hispanic female was referred for a speech and language evaluation by her preschool teacher. According to the child's teacher, the child and her family spoke English and Spanish. The child was screened initially for speech, language, and hearing in both languages. She did not respond to any of the items on the speech-language screening or to the pure-tone hearing screening. Consultation with the teacher revealed that the child was equally unresponsive to many of the teacher's requests and rarely interacted with her classmates. She was described as a very quiet, shy child. The teacher suspected a possible speech or hearing disorder.

Parental permission was requested for a speech, language, and hearing evaluation. The parents consented to the hearing evaluation but questioned the need for a speech and language evaluation. The hearing evaluation revealed normal hearing. As the school year progressed, the teacher's concerns increased. The teacher felt that she could not recommend this child for kindergarten, because she had not demonstrated many of the school's readiness skills expected of preschoolers. The parents were asked again to consent to a speech and language evaluation. The parents agreed reluctantly.

Given conflicting reports from the parents and teachers about the child's speech and language skills, it was important for the speech-language pathologist to ensure that the language samples gathered were representative of language functioning in a variety of settings, and that the approaches used to gather the samples were ecologically valid. Thus, an ethnographic assessment approach was used, according to Battle's (1997) guidelines. Also, a bilingual speech-language pathologist was consulted, to ensure that the evaluation and analysis procedures and conclusions were authentic. First, the child was observed over time in several environments. Speech and language samples were collected using videotape. A teacher-directed, small-group activity and a small-group free-play time were recorded at school. Free play with the parents was videotaped in a university speech and hearing clinic, and the parents videotaped free play at home with siblings. Second, the parents were asked to complete a case history questionnaire and to participate in an interview with an examiner at the university's speech and hearing clinic. The child's grandmother and one aunt also participated in the interview because they were frequent caretakers of the child. The child's teacher, teacher's aide, and physical education instructor were interviewed at the child's school. Third, the examiner and a graduate student clinician interacted with the child over two sessions in order to elicit language and play behaviors. Wordless books, toys, and stimuli from the English and Spanish versions of Preschool Language Scale (Zimmerman, Steiner, & Pond, 1992) were used.

The results of the assessment revealed that this child's speech and language skills were functional and appropriate in home settings. She sometimes used English and Spanish, interchangeably, as did all members of her family. There were times when a family member had difficulty understanding the child, but the child readily and effectively complied with requests for clarification. A family member interpreted the Spanish utterances for the examiner. The bilingual speech-language pathologist analyzed the language samples. Phonological, grammatical, semantic, and pragmatic aspects of language were found to be appropriate for the child's chronological age. However, in school, the child's verbal expressions were severely limited, and she did not respond to any of the language assessment tasks presented in English or Spanish in her school, in her classroom, or in the speech and hearing clinic.

Finally, her parents were instructed in giving the child the Preschool Language Scale, in Spanish and English, in their home, on separate days, with the speech-language pathologist present. The results gathered from this administration indicated that the child's speech was age-appropriate, but there were some weaknesses in vocabulary and grammar indicating a delay of one year. Based on these results, a home-based language intervention program was implemented. Also, the child's parents and grandmother were encouraged to come to school often and participate in reading stories to the class, go on field trips, and become parent helpers in order to help the child feel more comfortable in class. A reevaluation conducted four months later showed that the child is making gains with vocabulary in Spanish and English. Vocabulary gains include being able to give object descriptions and object functions, categorize concepts, identify colors, understand spatial concepts, and use pronouns correctly.

In truth, it cannot be said whether the gains shown in the postassessment actually result from growth in vocabulary and grammatical knowledge, or from increased familiarity with the school's climate and the nature of school-related tasks. What can be said, however, is that ecological assessment served to ease the fears and distrust of family members and satisfy the concerns of the teachers, as well as to create a functional language intervention plan for a four-year-old who was at risk for school failure.

CONCLUSION (REPRISE)

Both sociocultural and functional perspectives must be considered in shaping treatment outcomes. Decisions about treatment strategies, clinical activities, and clinical material selections are determined in accordance with environmental demands, individual abilities, and preferences and social traditions. To achieve a sociocultural and functional perspective, clinicians must recognize their clients' communication needs as reflective of their abilities, as well as their world experiences. What clients believe to be possible, useful, and important as multicultural and diverse individuals will have a direct impact on whether they reach their goals.

Critics and historians often view the concerto as the supreme synthesis of instrumental music. Analogously, desirable clinical outcomes represent the supreme synthesis of sociocultural and functional knowledge. Unfortunately, having made this assertion, the authors still cannot play the piano. But they hope they have led their reader to orchestrate their own sociocultural and functional perspectives.

Discussion Questions

1. In what ways will similarities and differences in the clinician's and client's macro-, meso-, and microcultures affect the clinical process?
2. What are the benefits of developing culturally appropriate functional goals?
3. How could Battle's 1997 guidelines be used to develop an evaluation protocol for a new client?
4. How could certain sociocultural variables influence the effectiveness of a treatment strategy designed to increase an adolescent's ability to follow complex directions in the school, home, and after-school work settings?
5. What are possible differences in the amount, clarity, and accuracy of information found in case histories taken from three different mothers whose children attend the same elementary school in a rural part of the country?

REFERENCES

American Speech-Language Hearing Association. (1997). *Preferred practice patterns for the profession of speech-language pathology*. Rockville, MD: Author.

Andrini, B. (1991). *Cooperative learning and mathematics*. San Juan Capistrano, CA: Resources for Teachers.

Banks, J.A., & Banks, C.A. (1997). *Multicultural education: Issues and perspectives* (3rd ed.). Needham Heights, MA: Allyn and Bacon.

Battle, D.E. (1997). Language and communication disorders in culturally and linguistically diverse children. In K.K. Bernstein & E. Tiegerman-Farber. *Language and communication disorders in children* (3rd ed.) (pp. 382–410). Needham Heights, MA: Allyn and Bacon.

Bauman, R., & Sherzer, J. (1989). *Explorations in the ethnography of speaking* (2nd ed.). New York: Cambridge University Press.

Cornett, B.S., & Chabon, S.S. (1988). *The clinical practice of speech-language pathology*. Columbus, OH: Merrill Publishers.

Crago, M.B. (1992). Ethnography and language socialization: A cross-cultural perspective. *Topics in Language Disorders, 12*, (3), 28–39.

Damico, J.S., & Hamayan, E.V. (1992). *Multicultural language intervention: Addressing cultural and linguistic diversity.* Chicago: Riverside Publishers.

Damico, J.S., Smith, M., & Augustine, L.E. (1996). Multicultural populations and language disorders. In M.D. Smith & J.S. Damico (Eds.), *Childhood language disorders* (pp. 272–299). New York: Thieme Medical Publishers.

Deshler, D.D., & Putnam, M.L. (1996). Learning disabilities in adolescents: A perspective. In D. Deshler, E. Ellis, & B.K. Lenz (Eds.). *Teaching adolescents with learning disabilities*, (2nd ed.) (pp. 1–6). Denver, CO: Love Pub. Co.

Dunn, L., & Dunn, L. (1997). *Peabody picture vocabulary test-III.* Circle Pine, MN: American Guidance Services Publishers.

Hammill, D.D., & Newcomer, P.L. (1988) *Test of language development-intermediate second edition.* Austin, TX: Pro-Ed.

Knapp, M.S., Thurnball, B.J., & Shields, P.M. (1990). New directions for educating the children of poverty. *Educational Leadership, 48*, (1), 4–8.

Kreb, R.A., & Wolf, K.E. (1997). *Successful operations in the treatment-outcomes-driven world of managed care*, Clinical Series 13. Rockville, MD: American Speech-Language Hearing Association.

Lenz, B.K., Schumaker, J.B., Deshler, D.D., & Beals, V.L. (1984). *The learning strategies curriculum: The word identification strategy.* Lawrence, KS: University of Kansas Institute for Research in Learning Disabilities.

Lynch, E.W., & Hanson, M.J. (1992). *Developing cross-cultural competence: A guide for working with young children and their families.* Baltimore: Paul H. Brookes Publishing Co.

McCormick, L. (1997). Ecological assessment and planning. In L. McCormick, D.F. Loeb, & R.L. Schiefelbusch (Eds.), *Supporting children with communication difficulties in inclusive settings* (pp. 223–256). Needham Heights, MA: Allyn and Bacon.

Nelson, N.W. (1998). *Childhood language disorders in context: Infancy through adolescence* (2nd ed.). Needham Heights, MA: Allyn and Bacon.

Oller, J.W. (1983). Some working ideas for language teaching. In J.W. Oller & P.W. Richard-Amato (Eds.). *Methods that work: A smorgasboard of ideas for language teachers* (pp. 3–19). Rowley, MA: Newbury House.

Parloff, M.B., Waskow, I.E., & Wolfe, B.E. (1978). Research on therapist variables in relation to process and outcome. In S.L. Garfield & A.E. Bergin (Eds.), *Handbook of psychotherapy and behavior change* (2nd ed.) (pp. 233–283). New York: John Wiley & Sons.

Pelligrini, A.D., Galda, L., & Rubin, D.L. (1984). Context in text: The development of oral and written language in two genres. *Child Development, 33*, 1549–1555.

Roberts, R.N. (1990). *Developing culturally competent programs for children with special needs.* Washington, DC: Georgetown University Child Development Center.

Roberts, S.D., & Hutchison, H.T. (1998). *Treatment outcomes: Making them work for you.* Paper presented at the 1998 ASHA Leadership in Service Delivery Conference, Tucson, AZ.

Romski, M.A., & Sevcik, R. (1996). Communication development of children with severe disabilities. In M.D. Smith & J.S. Damico (Eds.), *Childhood language disorders* (pp. 218–234). New York: Thieme Medical Publishers.

Saville-Troike, M. (1978). *A guide to culture in the classroom.* Washington, DC: National Clearinghouse for Bilingual Education.

Schumaker, J.B., Deshler, D.D., & Denton, P. (1984). *The learning strategies curriculum: The paraphrasing strategy*. Lawrence, KS: University of Kansas.

Semel, E., Wiig, E.H., & Secord, W. (1987). *Clinical evaluation of language fundamentals-revised*. New York: The Psychological Corporation, Harcourt Brace Jovanovich, Inc.

Silliman, E.R., & Wilkinson, L.C. (1991). *Communicating for learning classroom observation and collaboration*. Gaithersburg, MD: Aspen Publishers, Inc.

Silliman, E.R., & Wilkinson, L.C. (1994). Observation is more than looking. In G.P. Wallach & K.G. Butler (Eds.). *Language learning disabilities in school-age children and adolescents: Some principles and applications* (pp. 145–173). New York: Macmillan.

Tarulli, N.J. (1998). Using photography to enhance language and learning: A picture can encourage a thousand words. *Language, Speech and Hearing Services in Schools, 29*, (1): 54–57.

Taylor, O.L. (Unpublished paper). Clinical practice as a social occasion: An ethnographic model.

Taylor, O.L., Payne, K.T., & Anderson, N.B. (1987). Distinguishing between communication disorders and communication differences. *Seminars in Speech and Language, 8*, 415–427.

U.S. Department of Education. (1994). *National agenda for achieving better results for children and youth with serious emotional disturbance*. Prepared by The Chesapeake Institute, U.S. Department of Education, Office of Special Education and Rehabilitative Services, Office of Special Education Program. Washington, DC: U.S. Government Printing Office.

Wechsler, D. (1974). *Wechsler intelligence scale for children—revised (WISC-R).* New York: The Psychological Corporation.

Zimmerman, I.L., Steiner, V.G., & Pond, R.E. (1992). *Preschool language scale-3*. San Antonio, TX: The Psychological Corporation. Harcourt Brace Jovanovich, Inc.

SUGGESTED READINGS

Lynch, E., & Hanson, M. (1988). *Developing cross-cultural competencies: A guide for working with young children and their families*. Baltimore: Paul H. Brookes Publishing.

Mallory, B., & New, R. (1994). *Diversity and developmentally appropriate practices*. New York: Teachers College Press.

Payne, J. (1997). *Adult neurogenic language disorders: Assessment and treatment*. San Diego, CA: Singular Publishing Group.

Seymour, C., & Nober, F. (1998). *Introduction to communication disorders: A multicultural approach*. Woburn, MA: Butterworth-Heinermann.

Wallace, G. (1997). *Multicultural neurogenics. A resource for speech-language pathologists*. San Antonio, TX: Communication Skill Builders.

York, S. (1991). *Roots and wings: Affirming culture in early childhood programs*. St. Paul, MN: Redleaf Press.

Appendix 7–A Questions Regarding Cultural Factors, Family, and Community

GENERAL

1. What are the major stereotypes that you and others have about each cultural group?
2. To what extent and in what areas has the traditional culture of each minority group changed in contact with the dominant culture? In what areas has it been maintained?
3. To what extent do individuals possess knowledge of or exhibit characteristics of traditional groups?

FAMILY

1. Who is in a "family"? Who among these (or others) live in the house?
2. What is the hierarchy of authority in the family?
3. What are the rights and responsibilities of each family member? Do children have an obligation to work to help the family?
4. What are the functions and obligations of the family in the larger social unit?
5. What is the degree of solidarity or cohesiveness in the family?

THE LIFE CYCLE

1. What are the criteria for the definition of stages, periods, or transitions in life?
2. What are the attitudes, expectations, and behaviors toward individuals at different stages in the life cycle?
3. What behaviors are appropriate or unacceptable for children of various ages? How might these conflict with behaviors taught or encouraged in the school?
4. How is language related to the life cycle?
5. How is the age of children computed? What commemoration is made of the child's birth (if any) and when?

ROLES

1. What roles within the group are available to whom, and how are they acquired? Is education relevant to this acquisition?
2. Is language use important in the definition or social marking of roles?
3. Are there class differences in the expectations about child role attainment? Are they realistic?

INTERPERSONAL RELATIONSHIPS

1. How do people greet one another? What forms of address are used between people in various roles?
2. Do girls work and interact with boys? Is it proper?
3. How is deference shown?
4. How are insults expressed?
5. Who may disagree with whom? Under what circumstances?

COMMUNICATION

1. What languages, and varieties of each language, are used in the community? By whom? Where?
2. Which varieties are written? How widespread is knowledge of written forms?
3. What are the characteristics of "speaking well"? How do these relate to age, sex, context, or other social factors? What are the criteria for correctness?
4. What roles, attitudes, or personality traits are associated with particular ways of speaking?
5. What is considered "normal" speech behavior?
6. Is learning language a source of pride? Is developing bilingual competence considered an advantage or a handicap?
7. What gestures or postures have special significance or may be considered objectionable? What meaning is attached to making direct eye contact? To eye avoidance?
8. Who may talk to whom? When? Where? About what?

DECORUM AND DISCIPLINE

1. What counts as discipline in terms of the culture and what doesn't?
2. What behaviors are considered socially acceptable for students of different age and sex?
3. Who (or what) is considered responsible if a child misbehaves?
4. Who has authority over whom? To what extent can one person's will be imposed on another? By what means?
5. How is the behavior of children traditionally controlled, to what extent, and in what domains?
6. What is the role of language in social control? What is the significance of using the first versus the second language?

RELIGION

1. What is considered sacred and what secular?
2. What religious roles and authority are recognized in the community? What is the role of children in religious practices?
3. What taboos are there? What should not be discussed in school? What questions should not be asked? What student behaviors should not be required?

FOOD

1. What is eaten? In what order? How often?
2. What foods are favorites? What is taboo? What is typical?
3. What rules are observed during meals regarding age and sex roles within the family, the order for serving, seating, utensils used, and appropriate verbal formulas (e.g., how and if one may request, refuse, or thank)?
4. What social obligations are there with regard to food giving, preparation, reciprocity, and honoring people?
5. What relation does food have to health? What medicinal uses are made of food or categories of food?
6. What are the taboos or prescriptions associated with the handling, offering, or discarding of food?

DRESS AND PERSONAL APPEARANCE

1. What clothing is typical? What is worn for special occasions? What seasonal differences are considered appropriate?
2. How does dress differ for age, sex, and social class?
3. What restrictions are imposed for modesty?
4. What is the concept of beauty or attractiveness? What characteristics are most valued?
5. Does the color of dress have symbolic significance?

HISTORY AND TRADITIONS

1. What individuals and events in history are a source of pride for the group?
2. To what extent is knowledge of the group's history preserved? In what forms?
3. Do any ceremonies or festive occasions commemorate historical events?
4. How and to what extent does the group's knowledge of history coincide with or depart from scientific theories of creation, evolution, and historical development?
5. To what extent does the group identify with the history and traditions of their country of origin? What changes have taken place in the country of origin since the group or individuals emigrated?
6. For what reasons or under what circumstances did the group or individuals come to this country?

HOLIDAYS AND CELEBRATIONS

1. What holidays and celebrations are observed by the group and individuals? What is their purpose (e.g., political, seasonal, religious)?
2. Which are especially important for children and why?
3. What cultural values are they intended to inculcate?
4. Do parents and students know and understand school holidays and behavior appropriate for them?

EDUCATION

1. What is the purpose of education?

2. What methods for teaching and learning are used at home (e.g., modeling and imitation, didactic stories and proverbs, direct verbal instruction)? Do methods vary with the setting or according to what is being taught or learned?
3. What is the role of language in learning and teaching?
4. Is it appropriate for students to ask questions or volunteer information?
5. What constitutes a positive response by a teacher to a student?
6. How many years is it considered normal for children to go to school?
7. Are there different expectations by parents, teachers, and students with respect to different groups? In different subjects? For boys versus girls?
8. How are children with disabilities or special learning needs managed in the country of origin?
9. What are the family's expectations for their child's education and for the future?

WORK AND PLAY

1. What range of behaviors are considered "work" and what "play"?
2. What kinds of work are prestigious and why? Why is work valued?
3. Are there stereotypes about what a particular group will do?
4. What is the purpose of play?

TIME AND SPACE

1. What beliefs or values are associated with concepts of time? How important is punctuality? How important is speed of performance when taking a test?
2. Is control or prescriptive organization of children's time required (e.g., must homework be done before watching TV; is bedtime a scheduled event)?
3. What significance is associated with different directions or places (e.g., heaven is up, people are buried facing West)?

Source: Reprinted with permission from Saville-Troike, M. (1978). A Guide to Culture in the Classroom, Washington, D.C.: National Clearinghouse for Bilingual Education. http://www.ncbe.gwu.edu/ncbepubs/classics/culture/index.htm.

PART III

Looking Ahead: Perspectives on Our Future

The worlds of health care and education are not that far apart. Both sectors are experiencing wide-ranging reforms as services are scrutinized, dollars are rationed, and consumers are demanding specific outcomes. Alex Johnson and Lissa Power-deFur have agreed to "go out on a limb" and offer perspectives on current and continuing changes for professional practice in these broad areas. The author discusses ideas about a preferred (or "dream") future for speech-language pathologists versus a future that reflects more sobering trends in health and education settings.

More than 10 years ago, Larkins (1986) and Cole (1986) offered their perspectives on the future. Looking forward 10 years, Larkins (1986) said that four major trends would affect clinical practice:

1. changing demographics
2. the health care system's focus on cost-effectiveness and quality assessment
3. the changing roles of allied health professionals within the system
4. the continuing evolution of technology

A few names have changed, but these issues still drive our present and future (for education as well as health care).

Cole (1986) suggested that the viability of the speech-language pathology profession depends upon reaching the goal of becoming a "primary profession" and listed seven important characteristics.

1. Services provided are recognized widely as addressing an area of human functioning critical to well-being. These services are treated as essential components in the health services delivery system.

2. Members of the profession are recognized as experts in the area of human functioning for which they deliver services. They are primarily responsible for decisions concerning diagnosis and treatment of disorders in their area of expertise.
3. The profession accepts responsibility both for producing and applying new information in its own area of practice. It has a strong research component as well as a strong service delivery component.
4. The professionals are held directly accountable for the accuracy of their diagnoses and the effectiveness of their treatment programs.
5. The professionals are required by law to be licensed to practice. Standards for licensing and for ethical conduct are set and administered by the profession.
6. Services typically are covered in third-party reimbursement programs, both public and private.
7. The profession has both generalists and specialists. All have a basic, broad-based core of knowledge and skills that undergird more advanced specialization. (p. 41)

Compare Cole's suggested characteristics and the current status of the profession at the turn of the 21st century. How far have we come? How far yet to go? Compare Larkins's and Cole's projections and concerns with Johnson's discussions in different decades. The entire profession will benefit from some thoughtful consideration of these and many other perspectives. Our future depends on it.

REFERENCES

Cole, P. (1986). I want to shape my own future: How about you? *Asha 28* (9), 41–42.

Larkins, P. (1986). The challenges ahead for the practice of speech-language pathology. *Asha, 28* (9), 29–30.

CHAPTER 8

Speech-Language Pathology in Health Settings: A View of the Future

Alex Johnson

Objectives

- Identify factors from within the profession that are likely to affect the practice of speech-language pathology in the future.
- Identify external trends and factors that will affect the practice of speech-language pathology.
- Understand the importance and relevance of professional standards and standards programs (such as accreditation) to the future of speech-language pathology.
- Appreciate the difference between the "preferred" future and the "realistic" future.

INTRODUCTION

As one begins to think about the daunting challenge of writing about "the future" of speech-language pathology in health settings, several images come to mind including crystal balls, graphic depictions of "trends," and the ever-present (and perhaps overused) concept of "forces outside our control." This chapter represents thinking garnered from a variety of sources. In it, some of those external and internal factors that have affected and will affect the field of speech-language pathology are presented. Some suggestions are offered for those wishing to have an impact on the future course of the profession so as to produce the most optimal situation or the *preferred* future for practitioners and for consumers. This chapter concludes with a "philosophy" about the opportunities for integrating trends, the preferred future, and the need for patient focus.

The way in which a person perceives the future is affected by his or her current situation. How might an individual who is in mid-career, practicing in a successful hospital practice look at the future of speech-language pathology? How might a patient with a chronic communication disorder see the desired future of the field? What about the college professor? Or the entering graduate student? What about the individual considering beginning a doctoral program? What about an employer? Each of these persons, all key players in the world of speech-language pathology, probably looks at the future through a slightly different crystal ball. Each might see his or her *realistic* future (that which is most likely to occur) and the *preferred* future (that which is most desirable) in a unique light, because each brings a distinctive background and set of beliefs, attitudes, values, and desires to the discussion. In addition, each of those mentioned has certain "blind spots." These blind spots might reflect a lack of information ("I didn't know they changed the requirements"), a bias ("I don't think people with aphasia need *that* much treatment"), or even denial ("I don't think that Medicare will reduce services to my patients") about a key factor that could influence the future.

Hopefully, resources such as this book will help readers to avoid such blind spots as they move forward in the development of their career. Thus, the readers of this chapter are encouraged to take time to complete the exercise of looking toward a realistic future versus a preferred future. This approach will be useful to those wanting to understand their own beliefs and directions. By working to align the trends, forecasts, and changing practice patterns (realistic future) with their own desires, needs, and vision (preferred future), speech-language pathologists can modify what might occur. Speech-language pathologists have the potential to actually change the course of the realistic future, moving it in the direction of their preferences. Thus, attempting to steer "reality" toward a *vision* becomes a useful theme when considering the future.

SOURCES OF INFORMATION CONCERNING TRENDS AND THE FUTURE

The field of speech-language pathology is filled with various resources that members of the profession use to derive information to meet clinical, administrative, or research needs. The number of resources available continues to grow steadily. Journals, newsletters for special interest groups, texts, manuals, and a host of other products are continuously added to the pool of information available for speech-language pathologists to use. With the rapid growth of information on the Internet, the number of resources available to speech-language pathologists for purposes of planning and thinking about the future is somewhat overwhelming. These resources are not only abundant but also accessible in a timely and expedient (almost instantaneous) manner. Information that would have formerly taken weeks to access through interlibrary loan can be downloaded to a computer desktop in seconds or minutes. For a listing of useful links, please refer to Judith Kuster's web page (Kuster, 1998) http://www.mankato.msus.edu/dept/comdis/kuster2/welcome.html.

Based on the various sources of information available, several questions about the future of the profession are posed in this chapter:

- Changes in the organization and structure of service delivery—How will we do it?
- Changes in the content and scope of service delivery—What will we do?
- Changes in practice models and practitioners—Who will do it?

ORGANIZATION AND STRUCTURE OF SERVICE DELIVERY IN THE HEALTH CARE SETTING: HOW WILL WE PROVIDE SERVICES IN THE FUTURE?

Service delivery reflects the environment in which it is delivered. Services in hospitals look and feel different than services delivered in skilled-nursing facilities. Speech-language pathologists are expert at fitting into their work environment. Adaptability is a value that is initiated in graduate programs and is reinforced in clinical practicums and usually in early work experiences. Although speech-language pathologists come from a common educational experience, the roles that they play in various settings are diverse. A variety of general issues affecting how speech-language pathologists will provide services in the future are first considered.

Economic Factors

It is not by chance that the first factors selected here are economic factors that affect the practice of speech-language pathology. These are probably the chief external variables that mold and influence delivery models. From an economic perspective, Medicare, managed care, and fee-for-service care are areas that are likely to significantly affect medical speech-language pathology.

Medicare

At the time of this writing, the Medicare program (which has for many years reimbursed practitioners and facilities—hospitals, nursing homes, and outpatient clinics—for delivering services to patients with communication disorders) is undergoing sweeping changes. If fully implemented, these changes will reduce the degree to which clinicians and programs can be reimbursed for providing services to elderly patients with disorders of speech, language, and swallowing. This follows a period of rapid growth in direct service to the elderly population, especially those in skilled-nursing facilities. It is not definite at this time what all of the effects on the volume, type, and scope of services might be, but it is clear that it will be difficult for providers to receive favorable reimbursement for many of the services currently provided. This is likely to cause careful reconsideration of the commitment made by some providers, especially those from the for-profit sector, to patients with serious disorders of speech and language and those with dysphagia. A good review of Medicare changes being proposed for medical speech-language pathology settings was published in the *ASHA Leader* ("Medicare," 1998). New tests and tools for determining service eligibility are being developed, and it will be imperative that speech-language pathologists become knowledgable in administering them so that the needs of their patients can be brought to the forefront. For example, in the long-term care environment the Minimum Data Set (MDS) has been established as the protocol for assessment of all residents. At the time of this writing the final plans for other comprehensive tools have not been implemented, it is not feasible to know the specific effects or specific recommendations for dealing with them. However, it is likely that changes directed at limiting care, curbing abuses in overutilization of services, and controlling costs will create serious challenges for speech-language pathologists committed to serving elders in both inpatient and outpatient settings.

Managed Care

Managed care has become an established, yet vigorously debated, manner of service delivery. Observation of this development over recent years suggests that more effort has been put into the management of resources than into the advancement of patient care. Although the rapid growth in managed care enrollment seen in the early 1990s has slowed in many geographic areas, there has been considerable growth in the number of elderly persons who are shifting to managed care plans in some markets and reductions in others. These plans allow them to convert their Medicare insurance and provide what is thought to be a more comprehensive service. In most clinical settings, speech-language pathologists are seeing patients who are funded by a variety of different types of insurers, including several different managed care organizations. Many have their own guidelines and clinical pathways, which specify the nature and scope of services to be provided for a given diagnosis. Managed care organizations use a variety of strategies to control overutilization of services by their enrollees or members. These strategies include limiting covered diagnoses for evaluation and treatment, limiting the number of treatment sessions or services, and providing disincentives for referrals made by primary-care physicians to other providers such as speech-language pathologists. Such disincentives can include reducing the number of referrals from the managed care organization, reducing the financial return, or otherwise financially impacting the physician's practice.

Accompanying the expansion of managed care services in the past 10 years, there has been strong reaction from consumers. Recent media attention has focused on problems experienced by consumers in access and/or convenience of services, quality of services, range of services or providers available, and lack of attention to the "humane or compassionate" components of health care. Although the media are typically attracted to the most dramatic stories, one only has to attend the neighborhood barbecue to hear direct concerns being voiced by someone who had to wait for several weeks for an appointment or who had to drive for more than an hour to see the specialist who was "in network." At least one article (Peeno, 1998) in a popular magazine has focused specifically on the conflict between quality of life and cost controls inherent to managed care in a patient with a serious disorder of communication. See Chapter 1 in this text for more information about managed care.

Fee-for-Service Care

Predictions from the late 1980s and early1990s suggested the demise of fee-for-service care. However, recent curtailments in governmental programs (Medicare and Medicaid) and limitations imposed by some managed care organizations have provided an environment where some patients appear to be willing, if somewhat reluctantly, to fund some of their care by paying the provider directly. As the current trend in reduced insurance reimbursement for speech-language pathology services continues, it is likely that increased attention will be given to the very competitive fee-for-service market.

Professional Standards and Practices

Acceptable professional practices are derived from the various knowledge sources of the discipline and from a mutually agreed-upon set of standards of practice. The American Speech-Language-Hearing Association (ASHA), the major professional body influencing professional practice in speech-language pathology, provides standards for certification in speech-language pathology (ASHA, 1995), standards for organization and delivery of services (ASHA, 1995), and standards for accreditation of graduate programs. ASHA also provides a "Code of Ethics" (ASHA, 1994) and standards for the accreditation of continuing education providers in speech-language pathology and audiology. Currently, ASHA is in the process of developing standards for the recognition of two divergent groups—specialists in various clinical areas and speech-language pathology assistants.

The importance and influence of ASHA's governance and standards-setting bodies upon the conduct of professional services may be underestimated by the practitioner. ASHA, through consultation and deliberation with its various constituencies, establishes and promotes the standards for service delivery and education that guide the development of the profession. Vital areas addressed through the various standards and accreditation bodies associated with ASHA include questions such as the following:

- Is there a need for a clinical doctorate?
- What should the minimum continuing education requirements be for renewal of the ASHA Certificate of Clinical Competence in Speech-Language Pathology (CCC-SLP) (ASHA, 1993)?
- How should speech-language pathology assistants be selected, trained, and recognized? What should be the scope of their practice?
- What are minimum requirements for entry into independent practice?
- What clinical practicums are necessary?

- How should specialty and subspecialty areas with communication disorders be recognized?

As these questions (along with a myriad of others) are addressed, the practice of the profession will be defined for the next generation of speech-language pathologists and their patients. The influence of these policy decisions is of utmost importance to practitioners and consumers. Clearly, speech-language pathologists who wish to have a voice in their future should be sure to participate as fully as possible in the surveys and other studies conducted by ASHA. These communication approaches are designed to allow individuals to voice their opinions and provide valuable data about important issues.

Government

Another important defining influence in speech-language pathology is the area of federal, state, and local government. Rules, laws, and court opinion all influence practices within the profession. The areas that are defined and implemented by the government include some aspects of reimbursement, licensure, and state and national health reforms. In addition, governmental agencies (such as Veterans Administration; state hospitals and prisons; and the military) serve as the primary employer for many speech-language pathologists. General trends within government affect quality of care and employment.

Perhaps the most important governmental area having an impact upon practice is the area of licensing. At this time, most states have enacted licensure laws to define and control speech-language pathology practice. Regulations for licensure advance recognition of the profession and protect the public. In upcoming years, many existing licensure laws will be "opened" as part of an ongoing "sunset" review process. "Sunsetting" refers to mandated review of legislation over a specified period of time. Without such review and establishment of a rationale for continuing the law, the legislation is discontinued. Given the current legislative trend toward reducing government regulation, some licensure laws may be revoked or diminished. This possibility serves as a reminder of the continued importance of governmental advocacy by members of the profession. It also underscores the continued need for the ASHA Certificate of Clinical Competence (CCC), which serves as a national standard available to speech-language pathologists regardless of the legislative situation in a given state. It may be that in the future, the ASHA CCC will serve as the model for a singular national licensure bill.

Technology

The potential impact of technology on the future of clinical practice is significant. Most speech-language pathologists trained in the 1970s and 1980s have experienced dramatic shifts in the breadth and depth of their practice. Utilization of clinical instrumentation in the medical setting has become routine. Speech-language pathologists are involved in endoscopy, brain mapping, videofluoroscopy, and biofeedback. The availability of computer technology in most clinics and hospitals has afforded the opportunity to develop improved information systems for maintaining patient files, measuring progress and outcomes, and communicating among professionals. The advent and widespread use of the Internet as a source of communication and information has dramatically changed access to resources that were only dreams 5 or 10 years ago. The various information sources on the Internet are beginning to be widely used by consumers in addition to providing speed and efficiency for clinicians. Condition-specific information, referral sources, support groups, and chat rooms are increasingly available. As with television, radio, and the print media, there is the potential for tremendous misinformation on the Internet. Because virtually anyone with a computer and a modem can submit information to the Internet, the issues of accuracy and appropriateness will be important factors for both clinicians and their patients as new technology applications emerge.

In addition to the information sources available using computer technologies, the important question regarding the interactive capabilities of the computer to enhance therapy must be considered. One vendor (Scientific Research Corporation) has developed a specific auditory-processing therapy program that is delivered to the patient via computer; communications via the Internet are used to provide daily adjustments in the stimuli and content of the program. Another group (Language Care Centers Inc.) has integrated existing computer technology into a defined therapy program and augmentative communication system for persons with chronic aphasia. These two developments are likely precursors to a number of new technologies for people with other types of speech and language problems. As such technologies emerge, services may be made accessible to new populations of persons with communicative disorders. However, the potential for misapplication of these technologies will create new challenges in the ethical and reimbursement arenas.

Technology is changing rapidly. Computers are more affordable and faster. Scanners, fax machines, high-speed modems, and multimedia all contribute to the possibility that future generations of clinicians will use technology routinely to add dimensions to care that we have not yet begun to think about. For example, the new interactive medium of telemedicine is being promoted as an affordable manner of obtaining consultation, especially for patients in rural or remote settings. A model for delivering medical speech-language pathology consultative and treatment services via telemedicine technology has been described by Duffy, Werven, and Aronson (1997). Additional background information regarding telehealth technology has been discussed by Goldberg (1997).

Consumer Expectations and Perceptions

Consumer expectations is perhaps the most influential factor affecting the future of speech-language pathology in the health care setting. Consumers are now vital participants in every aspect of their own health care. The patient of the 1990s is likely to "shop" for the provider who can deliver the best service (as defined by the patient), in the most convenient location, in the most economical manner. In addition, consumers have developed more skepticism about health care than ever before. They expect to participate in all decisions, and they expect outcomes that are observable and affect the quality of their life. Not only do these factors shape the economics of speech-language pathology practice, but they increase a demand for new resources and new models of service delivery that allow for involvement of patients in decision making at every level of care and extend services to the family system as well as the patient.

A second aspect of increased consumer focus has to do with the demand for services and support beyond the process of direct intervention or therapy. As in many areas of health care, there is growth in the number of support groups available for people with speech, language, and swallowing disorders. Patients seem to be recognizing the implications of the chronicity of some communication disorders. They are expressing interest in access to services that emphasize healthy communication and participation in human interactions beyond the framework typically afforded in standard treatment paradigms focused at the level of the patient's impairment. Examples of new, consumer-driven organizations include the National Aphasia Association, the National Stuttering Project, the National Spasmodic Dysphonia Association, and many others. Again, the Internet provides an important resource for transmitting information to consumers and provides important opportunities for communication among providers. Hundreds of electronic bulletin boards and chat rooms have already been developed for persons with various disabilities. These mechanisms of interaction and communication, with a focus toward communication and interaction among consumers, are likely to continue to expand, as more individuals become participants in cyberspace. The unique features of the Internet allow for affordable and direct interaction among persons who are homebound or have other limitations. The many possibilities afforded by this important medium for persons with communication disorders are only beginning to be realized. As technologies and efficiencies of electronic communication are advanced, so are the benefits to consumers. It is important for practitioners to realize the potential for expanding opportunities for patient support, information sharing, and even direct treatment.

Forecast: Impact of Environmental Influences on Future Practice

The common factor among the issues discussed above is that they are somewhat external to the content and style of practice. That is, they affect speech-language pathology practice because of their importance to health care delivery and the culture at large. What will be their effect on the way speech-language pathologists will practice their profession in the future? The following considerations are offered as the direction of the *realistic* future:

- There will be continued pressure to reduce costs; payers and referral sources will seek ways to limit those factors that most directly affect cost—length of time in treatment and number of visits—as well as those that have little proven benefit.
- Two major payers of health care speech-language pathology services—Medicare and managed care organizations—will continue to attempt to influence the content of care as well as its cost. Referral guidelines will become more readily available and used regularly. Clinical pathways will be used to improve service efficiency, to provide a focus to treatment, and to increase communication among

the core team. However, these tools will also be used to *limit* service utilization. Expanded networks of care, with large databases, will allow standardization of practice. National benchmarking data regarding services in speech-language pathology such as ASHA's NOMS (1998) will be commonly used to compare programs and practitioners.

- Institutions will work diligently to attract the fee-for-service market. Discounts, free services, and other incentives will be used to bring patients who pay cash into the institution in order to compensate for shrinking reimbursement from governmental and private insurance sources. Clearly, a challenge of the future will be balancing resources to meet needs of patients who are enrolled in managed care programs and those who have more resources for payment.
- Standards will be developed to allow recognition of additional subspecialty areas within speech-language pathology. In addition, revisions in the requirements for the Certificate of Clinical Competence in Speech-Language Pathology (CCC-SLP) will reflect new trends and practices. This may force changes in the areas of graduate education (curricula and degree requirements), clinical experience (graduate practicuum), continuing education (mandated vs. optional), and the clinical fellowship year (length, scope, content).
- The government at every level will continue to influence practice and service delivery. As reimbursement structures change, services will be less readily available, especially to those most in need—the elderly and young children with severe health problems. In addition, state governments will resist implementation of changes in state licensure laws, even when the prevailing logic or expertise suggests that such changes would elevate practice standards.
- Speech-language pathologists will use the Internet to increase the range and scope of services. Computer technology will become more user-friendly, so that patients can reinforce therapy at home and can use therapy materials outside the clinic. Home-based computer therapy will also become more interactive, thereby providing more feedback to patients and clinicians and allowing the possibility for on-line modifications in stimuli based on a patient's accuracy and efficiency in responding.
- Speech-language pathologists will continue to develop and expand aspects of telemedicine as an alternative method of service delivery.

This will be attractive to referral sources and patients who live long distances from major medical centers.

- New networks and databases will allow for integration of large data sets of information. This information will be useful for planning services, as well as for program evaluation.
- Consumers will continue to demand services of very high quality, despite shrinking resources to support care. The lack of available resources to meet consumer demand will continue to create tensions between health institutions, providers, and patients. Clinicians and program directors will continue to struggle with ways to do more with less. In fact, the competition among providers will increase as institutions vie for those patients who have favorable reimbursement plans.
- Consumers will be most attracted to clinics and hospitals that provide the full range of services and assist with management of their communication disorder beyond the therapy session. Support groups, Internet access, counseling, and other services will be desirable. In addition, patients with multiple needs will pursue providers who offer access to all the services that they need. Programs that provide only one service, such as speech-language pathology, will find it difficult to compete as single providers.

THE SCOPE AND CONTENT OF SERVICE DELIVERY: WHAT WILL WE DO IN THE FUTURE?

The scope of speech-language pathology service delivery has expanded significantly since the early part of the 20th century. In the health care setting, speech-language pathologists have emerged as providers who consult, educate other professionals, provide direct evaluation and treatment, and counsel patients and families. Furthermore, the expertise of speech-language pathologists is recognized in differential diagnosis and management of conditions that result from a variety of physical, cognitive, developmental, genetic, and psychological conditions affecting communication. In the past 15 years, the scope of practice in medical speech-language pathology in acute and rehabilitative care has been extended to a number of clinical areas including dysphagia (Logemann, 1998), traumatic brain injury rehabilitation (Ylvisaker & Szekeres, 1994), augmentative communication (Yorkston, 1992), and right-hemisphere syndromes

(Tompkins, 1995). Each of these "new" areas of practice has provided a demand for additional levels of skill, knowledge, education, and supervision. In additon, new technologies and new opportunities for collaboration have resulted from these areas of advanced practice. In the long-term care setting, the role of speech-language pathologists has been expanded to include responsibilities for the nutritional management of patients with chronic conditions, assessment and rehabilitation of patients with cognitive-linguistic disturbance, and ensuring that patients are meeting their full social-interaction potential. In these settings, many speech-language pathologists are also taking on responsibilities as case managers, program supervisors, and directors; in these positions, they are frequently supervising members of other professions.

Content

The major areas of practice in the current medical speech-language pathology setting include neurogenic communication disorders, voice disorders, acute care (inpatient) speech-language pathology, pediatric communication disorders, dysphagia, and interdisciplinary rehabilitative care in subacute and long-term care settings. Several other areas of practice are emphasized in some specialized medical centers; however, those listed here are the most common. Although it is beyond the scope of this chapter to explore these areas in detail, it is important to highlight the key areas of current emphasis and change.

Dysphagia

Perhaps no area of practice in the field of speech-language pathology has grown as much or gained such a powerful voice as that of swallowing disorders in the health care setting. Health institutions and physicians have accepted speech-language pathologists in the area of diagnosis and management of this condition. In hospitals and skilled-nursing facilities, speech-language pathologists are consulted on a regular basis for patients with problems in deglutition, regardless of their communicative status. Some clinicians in hospital settings are frustrated because they no longer receive referrals to treat patients with neurologic communication disorders, but they are routinely consulted to see those with dysphagia. On the other hand, some clinicians have attributed the survival of speech-language pathology in adult health care settings to the rapid growth of dysphagia evaluation and treatment services. Regardless of one's position on this issue, it is obvious that the increased attention to practice in this area has expanded speech-language pathologists' roles in areas that extend beyond traditional speech and language services. In the future, the continued expansion of the services and role of speech-language pathologists in providing services to those with dysphagia is likely.

Neurogenic Communication Disorders

Several factors are affecting service to patients with diseases of the nervous system. Cutbacks in funding for services are forcing severe limitations on access to care. For example, despite evidence that some stroke patients can benefit from extended language rehabilitation programs, many insurance companies and managed care organizations have placed strict limitations on the extent of service available for persons with aphasia. In addition, for some patients with neurodegenerative diseases, payment for services is denied because the payer perceives that the patient lacks rehabilitation potential. Even when speech-language pathology services have the potential to significantly affect the patient's quality of life or nutrition, services may be denied. The implementation of the Balanced Budget Act of 1997 (U.S. Government, 1977) is one example of an attempt to cut costs which when fully implemented would cut costs to patients in long term care settings.

Another dimension of care that is increasingly emphasized by providers and consumers (but not payers) is a growing emphasis on the psychosocial aspects of communication and functioning in the culture. Some authors suggest that this emphasis should replace or at least reduce the emphasis on more traditional linguistic, cognitive, and behavioral emphases in treatment. Petheram and Parr (1998) provide a perspective regarding this tension among aphasiologists.

Finally, the aforementioned developments in the consumer advocacy and support area are quite obvious in the neurogenics area. Support groups, on-line resources, and consumer organizations are emerging rapidly.

Voice Disorders

New technologies for assessment and treatment of voice disorders have expanded rapidly over the past 15 years. Sophisticated voice laboratories with extensive capabilities for imaging the larynx and related structures are available in most major centers. Collaborative practice models between speech-language pathologists and otolaryngologists are common. In addition, new treatments for patients with head and neck cancer and those with other voice disorders are emerging at a rapid pace.

Acute Care Speech-Language Pathology

In major hospital settings, speech-language pathologists provide bedside consultative services for patients with acute medical problems. Silbergleit and Basha (1998) have described the role of the speech-language pathologist in the intensive care setting, with a focus on service to those patients who are ventilator dependent or who have tracheotomies. In addition, the role of speech-language pathologists in language testing with patients experiencing hyperacute stroke has been described by Johnson, Valachovic, and George (1998). Valachovic, Smith, Elisevich, Jacobson, and Fisk (1998) have described language mapping in the operating room as a function of the speech-language pathologist during neurosurgical procedures for management of epilepsy or brain tumors. These reports suggest that the role of speech-language pathologists in acute care has moved toward a high-tech role, collaborating with physicians and nurses in achieving optimal outcomes for patients in the most acute stage of their illnesses.

Pediatric Communication Disorders

Hospital and clinic-based services for children are covered by payers with decreasing frequency. Insurers often state that the needs of these children should be met within the educational system. However, many speech-language pathologists are increasing their attention toward children who are medically fragile. Communication and swallowing services for high-risk neonates is a relatively new area of practice. Services for hospitalized children who are medically fragile or acutely ill also continue to be a high priority in some health care settings.

Rehabilitative and Long-Term Care Services

The number and length of postacute rehabilitation stays have decreased with a trend toward rapid enrollment in outpatient care. In addition, speech-language pathologists have witnessed a rapid expansion of nursing home, extended-care, and home care services. A current threat to these services, especially for patients in long-term settings, is the change in payment for rehabilitation by the Medicare program. Prospective payment plans and payment caps are expected to curtail services to the elderly patient in long-term care. The impact of these cuts on the health and quality of life of institutionalized elders, as well as the impact on employment of clinicians may be quite serious. Many rehabilitation companies who employ large numbers of speech-language pathologists are reorganizing and downsizing in order to cut financial losses. Fewer professionals may be employed to provide services to patients in nursing homes and subacute rehabilitation settings. At the same time, services by speech-language pathologists in home settings are increasing (Tonkovich, 1998). The obvious benefit of home-based service is its accessibility to patients who are too weak or impaired to travel to the clinic, but yet do not require advanced medical and nursing care. Speech-language pathologists in all subacute settings are likely to need skills in providing direct service to patients and in supervising other individuals who deliver services to patients.

Forecast: Clinical and Professional Influences on Future Practice

Just as the environmental trends discussed in the first portion of this chapter are likely to have an effect on speech-language pathology practice, so will those factors that are more directly tied to the content of service delivery. Some likely trends include the following:

- In health care settings, those areas of practice most directly linked to the overall health and functional outcomes of the patient will receive the most emphasis. Conversely, areas that are likely to provide subtle behavioral change or less substantial benefit will be eliminated or at least reduced.
- Technologies that advance care, especially those with proven functional benefit, are likely to be improved and developed. Thus, speech-language pathologists will need even more skill in using these technologies. This has obvious implications for graduate and continuing education models, as well as standards-setting bodies.
- Speech-language pathologists in some medical settings will continue to be extended into roles that emphasize their knowledge and expertise in the function of the upper-aerodigestive tract in swallowing and respiratory functions as well as in speech and voice production.

- Speech-language pathologists will need to develop new service structures and models to serve patients who are most severely impaired and those with chronic neurologic conditions. Traditional payers will probably not fund services for the full scope of these patients' needs. Speech-language pathologists will need to use a variety of professional and community resources to achieve the best outcomes for their patients. Opportunities (and challenges) to collaborate with voluntary organizations as well as consumer groups must be addressed to ensure services of the highest quality.
- Clinicians will be called upon to provide more counseling and psychotherapeutic services to patients as they move through the continuum of care. Given the current attention to quality-of-life issues (see Frattali, 1998; Sarno, 1997), patients are likely to expect increased attention to long-term adjustment to their communicative problems. It will be important to teach families and patients principles of self-therapy, use of nontraditional resources, and self-empowerment skills as funding is reduced for long-term rehabilitation services.

CHANGES IN PRACTICE MODELS AND PRACTITIONERS: WHO WILL DO IT?

As we look to the future, the question of *who* will be doing the work in the field of human communicative disorders must receive some attention. Speech-language pathologists' colleagues in audiology have recently selected the doctoral level as the primary entry into clinical practice. This represents, for the first time in the history of the two professions, a divergence in the entry-level academic and clinical preparation for practice. At this time, there does not appear to be a demand for raising the academic standards within the speech-language pathology profession to the doctoral level. In fact, at the same time that the ASHA Standards Council has approved the doctoral level for audiology practice (ASHA, 1997), they are developing standards of practice for support persons in speech-language pathology. The roles and responsibilities of speech-language assistants have been under discussion for some time. However, the demand from the marketplace for more services at a reduced cost has driven the issue ahead. In certain settings and geographic regions, shortages of speech-language pathologists have increased this demand. Many speech-language pathologists in health settings are resisting the movement toward using support-level practitioners. It is likely that there will be continued debate on this topic.

Although the future academic degree requirements for practice in speech-language pathology are not clearly in place, it is clear that in medical settings a new brand of practitioner is emerging—the clinical specialist. For some time, various interest groups within ASHA and within specific work settings have been developing competencies for various types of advanced practice. ASHA has approved the development of a mechanism for the recognition of specialists, and a number of groups are in the process of applying for this recognition. For example, the Special Interest Division for Fluency Disorders (Division 4) has recently been approved to award specialization in the area of stuttering and related disorders. A related organization, the American Academy of Neurologic Communication Disorders and Sciences, has already developed and is awarding certification in the adult and child neurologic areas. While it is too early to estimate the numbers of practitioners who will receive certification or recognition as specialists, it is clear that this growing movement will have an effect on practice in the future.

Issues in Education and Research

The academic world has primary responsibility for the preparation of new speech-language pathologists. Beginning with the selection process for admission to graduate education and continuing through academic and clinical experiences, the mission of academe is to develop the speech-language pathologist for the future. Although the roles of the speech-language pathologist to be developed by university programs include clinician, teacher, and researcher, most individuals enrolled in academic programs choose to emphasize the role of clinicians as they advance in their careers. Currently, only a small number of students pursue doctoral education beyond their clinical preparation as a step toward a career in research, university teaching, or advanced clinical practice. In the next decade, many university programs will face the retirement of experienced faculty. There is likely to be a shortage of personnel with doctorates to fill these academic positions. Thus, a major issue for the profession in the future is how to provide adequate preparation for a growing number of clinical speech-language pathologists with a shrinking number of doctoral-level personnel (Wilson, 1998)?

The fact that the number of doctoral-level professionals is shrinking raises an equally important issue with regard to the future of research. How will the profession advance in knowledge if there are not enough well-prepared scientists within the field to engage in this vital work? Because the profession is knowledge based, it is essential that new information about the causes, effects, treatments, and technologies that affect speech, language, and swallowing be available. Recently, ASHA leaders and university personnel have begun to discuss the shortage of doctoral-level personnel. It is likely (and imperative) that clinical practitioners, employers, and consumers will begin to participate in the discussion. Opportunities exist to remove barriers that limit the numbers of individuals who choose an academic or scientific career path. In addition, we should explore potential for increased and more productive interaction among scholars and practitioners.

Forecast: Personnel Issues

The following trends among speech-language pathology personnel are likely:

- There will be increased awareness by consumers of individuals with special expertise and interest in their condition. Some consumers will demand treatment by these specialists.
- There will be increased recognition within the profession and among referral sources of specialists who might be able to provide advanced levels of consultation or technical expertise.
- The identification and recognition of layers of specialization may produce increased competition among providers holding various levels of recognized expertise.
- There will be a demand for the development of the identity and role of the general clinician in speech-language pathology. The well-prepared generalist may be a very desirable professional in organizations serving large numbers of patients and diverse populations.
- At the same time, the development of different categories of professionals within speech-language pathology may cause some confusion

among employers and payers when making decisions about hiring or payment for some services.

- There will be an opportunity and probably a significant demand for new levels of cooperation and communication among various speech-language pathology providers. Consultative arrangements among generalists and specialists will emerge. In addition, specialists will need to develop new skills in communicating effectively, efficiently, and respectfully with their generalist colleagues. Regardless of setting, all speech-language pathologists must develop a high degree of teaming skills with individuals in other professions.
- As the number of individuals prepared to function as speech-language pathology assistants grows, speech-language pathologists will need to develop tools and models for providing services to patients through others. In addition, new skills in the supervision of paraprofessionals will be required. Many clinicians will need special preparation to function effectively in this new supervisory role.
- University programs will begin to experience a major shortage in the availability of doctoral-level personnel for academic and research appointments. New roles for master's-level instructors are likely to be developed. Incentives for improved collaboration among practitioners and researchers will emerge so that scientific work can advance knowledge and practice. Models for collaboration among universities, development of programs in distance learning, and exploration of additional training roles for nonacademic clinical settings will also be explored as solutions to personnel shortages in academe.

CONCLUSION

This chapter attempts to capture some of the factors that will define the future of speech-language pathology. Members of the profession should all work to minimize trends that could reduce funding for services, negatively affect training or practice, or eliminate vital aspects of patient care. Conversely, speech-language pathologists should work to ensure that key trends that could benefit care and benefit the professionals who serve those in need will become real.

The concepts of *realistic* and *preferred* futures were discussed earlier in this chapter. Every clinician has the opportunity to participate in steering reality toward their preferred vision of what the future should be. While shrinking resources in health care may be evident for the next several years, professionals can and should use this time to explore new models of service delivery in health settings with an emphasis on the development of new technologies and models of collaboration. This is essential to the survival of the speech-language pathologist's role as health care provider for persons with communication and swallowing disorders. Although collaboration with other professions can be challenging and at times threatening, the possibilities afforded through shared knowledge and equitable cooperation should not be ignored. Similarly, barriers to advancement within the profession should not be ignored. Cooperation among practitioners across the health care continuum and in university settings can offer solutions to current problems within the clinical, academic, and research environments. Consider the benefit of integrated teaching, clinical training, and research sites designed to provide services across patient demographic and disability groups. Collaboration in such a setting would afford opportunities across disciplines for practitioners and researchers, as well as students.

We are living and working in an era of great change in health care. Hopefully, the ultimate benefit of so much change and tension will be improved care and advancement in knowledge. The threats of reduced funding and organizational restructuring will probably force a new level of adaptability and creativity among providers in every profession, including speech-language pathology. If individual clinicians and their organizations can use the resources available to continue to produce good outcomes, the existing potential for a better future can be realized. Despite the threats that exist in the current environment, speech-language pathologists should be optimistic about the opportunities that will emerge and the ongoing contribution that members of the profession can make to persons who urgently need their services and care.

Discussion Questions

1. What is the difference between your preferred future and your realistic future? What can you do to minimize the difference?
2. What external issues identified in the chapter might have the most striking effect on the practice of speech-language pathology? Do you agree or disagree with the projections offered in the chapter? Why?
3. How has the role of the consumer of speech-language pathology services changed in the past 20 years? What impact will this change have on future practice?
4. What are the threats and opportunities afforded in each of the following clinical practice areas:
   - dysphagia
   - neurologic communication disorders

- pediatric communication disorders
- voice disorders

5. What are the current trends regarding practice specialization? How will the growth of specialization affect the practice of speech-language pathology in the future?

REFERENCES

American Speech-Language-Hearing Association. (1993). *Standards and implementation for the certificate of clinical competence in speech-language pathology. ASHA Desk Reference.* Rockville, MD: Author.

American Speech-Language-Hearing Association. (1994). Code of ethics. *Asha, 36* (Suppl. 13), 1–2.

American Speech-Language-Hearing Association. (1998). Standards for certification in audiology.

American Speech-Language-Hearing Association. (1995). Standards for professional service programs in audiology and speech-language pathology. *ASHA Desk Reference.* Rockville, MD: Author.

American Speech-Language-Hearing Association. (1998). National Outcomes Measurement Systems (NOMS); Gaining support of staff and administration. Presentation at Annual ASHA Convention. ASHA (1998). San Antonio, TX.

Duffy, J.R., Werven, G.W., & Aronson, A.E. (1997). Telemedicine and the diagnosis of speech and language disorders. *Mayo Clinic Proceedings, 72* (12), 1116–1122..

Frattali, C. (1998). Measuring modality-specific behaviors, functional abilities, and quality of life. In C. Frattali (Ed.), *Measuring outcomes in speech-language pathology* (pp. 55–88). New York: Thieme Medical Publishers.

Goldberg, B. (1997, Fall). Linking up with telehealth. *Asha, 39* (4), 26–31.

Johnson, A.F., Valachovic, A.M., & George, K.P. (1998). Speech-language pathology in the acute care setting: A consultative approach. In A. Johnson & B. Jacobson (Eds.), *Medical speech-language pathology: A practitioner's guide* (pp. 96–130). New York: Thieme Medical Publishers.

Kuster, J. *Net connections for communications disorders and sciences*. Mankato, MN: Mankato State University.

Logemann, J. (1998). *Evaluation and treatment of swallowing disorders* (2nd ed.). Austin, TX: Pro-Ed.

Medicare: How the new payment systems will affect you. (1998, September 8). *Asha Leader Extra*, *3* (17).

Peeno, L. (1997, March 3). What is the value of a voice? *US News & World Report*, 40–46.

Petheram, B., & Parr, S. (1998). Diversity in aphasiology: Crisis or increasing competence? *Aphasiology, 12,* 435–487.

Sarno, M.T. (1997). Quality of life in aphasia in the first post-stroke year. *Aphasiology, 11*, 665–680.

Silbergleit, A.K., & Basha, M.A. (1998). Speech-language pathology in the intensive care unit. In A. Johnson & B. Jacobson (Eds.), *Medical speech-language pathology: A practitioner's guide* (pp. 65–94). New York: Thieme Medical Publishers.

Tompkins, C. (1995). *Right hemisphere communication disorders: Theory and management.* San Diego, CA: Singular Publishing Group.

Tonkovich, J.D. (1998). Management of communicative disorders in non-acute settings: Home care, hospice, SNF. In A. Johnson & B. Jacobsen (Eds.) Medical Speech-Language Pathology. New York: Thieme.

United States Government. (1997). Balanced Budget Act of 1997.

Valachovic, A.M., Smith, B., Elisevich, K., Jacobson. G., & Fisk, J. (1998). Language and its management in the surgical epilepsy unit. In A. Johnson & B. Jacobson (Eds.), *Medical speech-language pathology: A practitioner's guide* (pp. 425–466). New York: Thieme Medical Publishers.

Wilcox, K.A. (1998). Replacing the professorate: Perspectives from a doctoral program. Proceedings of the Annual Meeting of the Council of Graduate Programs in Communication Sciences & Disorders.

Ylvisaker, M., & Szekeres, S. (1994). Management of the patient with closed head injury. In R. Chapey (Ed.), *Language intervention strategies in adult aphasia* (3rd ed.) (pp. 546–567). Baltimore: Williams & Wilkins.

Yorkston K. (1992). *Augmentative communication in the medical setting.* Tucson, AZ: Communication Skill Builders.

SUGGESTED READINGS

Brooks, G.B., & Gonzalez Rothi, L.J. Why specialty recognition? *ASHA. 39 (4): 14–5, 1997 Fall.* 98003838 *Complete Reference.*

Butler, K. Research and practice in the 21st century. *ASHA. 38 (4): 9, 1996 Fall.* 97075545 *Complete Reference.*

deFur, L.P., & Kellum, G. Designing a future *ASHA. 39 (4): 12, 1997 Fall.* 98003837 *Complete Reference.*

Geffner, D. Growing the field. Who will teach future generations? *ASHA. 39 (3): 37–42, 1997 Summer.* 97385903 *Complete Reference.*

Guadagnoli, E., & McNeil, B.J. Outcomes Research: Hope for the future or the latest rage? *Inquiry 31*: 14–24 (1994).

Kimbarow, M.L. Ahead of the curve. Improving service with speech-language pathology assistants. *ASHA. 39 (4): 41–4, 1997 Fall.* 98003842 *Complete Reference.*

Lubker, B.B. Epidemiology: An essential science for speech-language pathology and audiology [published erratum appears in J Commun Disord 1998 Mar–Apr; 31 (2):

195]. *Journal of Communication Disorders. 30 (4): 251–65; quiz 265–7, 1997 Jul-Aug.* 97352080 *Abstract. Complete Reference.*

Pichanton, A. Clinical Service Delivery Return. In A. Johnson and B. Jacobson (Ed.) *Medical speech-language pathology: A practitioner's guide* (pp. 425–466). New York: Thieme Medical Publishers.

Terrizzi A., Steckol, K.F. Is the undergraduate major still viable? *ASHA. 40 (1): 10–1, 1998 Winter.* 98120131 *Complete Reference.*

Uffen E. Where the jobs are. Keeping an eye on the future. *ASHA. 40 (1): 24–8, 1998 Winter.* 98120133 *Complete Reference.*

CHAPTER 9

Predicting the Future of Speech-Language Pathology in Public Schools

Lissa Power-deFur

We cannot know the future with certainty, but we can develop reasonable expectations of what is likely to happen.

—Gilbert Herer

Objectives

- Understand how a review of emerging trends within the profession and in the society at large can enable the learner to anticipate the future.
- Identify four to five anticipated future issues influencing school-based speech-language pathologists.
- Identify five strategies they can implement to better prepare themselves for possible future events.

INTRODUCTION

Predict the future? Given the demands of our day-to-day responsibilities, it seems overwhelming to consider predicting the future. Besides, it is just going to happen anyway, and one person cannot make a difference. So, why bother?

Futurists—those professionals who study, think about, and plan for the future—agree that there is no way to know what will happen in the future. However, they also point out that by studying the past and the present we *can* forecast possible or probable future events (World Future Society, 1993). By thinking and planning ahead, it is possible to have some influence over the future. Such study enables us to mitigate the consequences of potential difficult changes and be ready to capitalize on positive changes. As James Gelatt said: "Simply put, we have three choices. Let the future happen, and try to adjust; seek to anticipate what may transpire, and chart a course accordingly; or choose a future you want, and work to make it happen" (1994).

While serving as president of the American Speech-Language-Hearing Association (ASHA) in 1989, Gilbert Herer advised association members and leaders to pursue futures study. He noted that "such study . . . provides a basis for strategic planning and control" (Herer, 1989). Futures study begins by scanning internal and external factors that may influence the profession of speech-language pathology. These scans allow for identification of emerging trends and anticipation of future possibilities. It is then possible to identify strategies that may influence the effect of these future possibilities on our profession, our discipline, and our consumers.

This chapter scans those internal and external factors associated with speech-language pathology in public schools, addressing such factors as educational reform, finance, demographics, and advances in technology. The implications for future practice are discussed, and strategies are identified so that speech-language pathologist can position themselves for the future.

EDUCATIONAL REFORM

Academic Standards

Montgomery and Herer collaborated to develop a tutorial for public school personnel on the importance of futures thinking. They noted: "Education will be the major public agenda item and will be viewed as key to our economic growth" (1994). They certainly predicted accurately! Public education is undergoing numerous reforms. Widespread concern regarding the status of public education had its beginning in the 1980s. In 1988, *The Futurist*, a publication of the World Future Society, published an article about the future of public education by M.J. Cetron. Cetron cautioned: "The class of 2000, and their schools, face educational demands far beyond those of their parents' generation. And unless they can meet those demands successfully, the United States could be nearing its last days as a world power" (Cetron, 1990). This prediction of the future sounds extreme, but it represents the concerns Americans had with public education throughout the 1990s. Beginning with the landmark report, *A Nation at*

Risk, Americans spent more than a decade belaboring the quality of the nation's schools. Americans consistently gave the nation's schools a *C*, yet graded their child's school higher (Elam, Rose, & Gallup, 1994). Educators were told that the skill requirements needed for the workforce were not those that schools were teaching. The economic impact of the high dropout rate, high illiteracy rate, and shortage of qualified workers for business and industry were further touted as reasons for educational reform.

Americans' focus on local control of public education prevented efforts to establish a national set of education standards, which is found in most other industrialized countries. However, by the end of the 20th century, all states have established standards in the core content areas of English/language arts, mathematics, science, history and the social sciences (McLaughlin, Nolet, Rhim, & Henderson, 1999). Standards identify expectations for all students at each grade level and in each content area. Curriculum development at the state and local levels is following standard settings. Groups of educators work to develop the day-to-day instructional applications to ensure that students meet the standards. The Individuals with Disabilities Education Act (IDEA) of 1997 also emphasizes the importance of standards. IDEA presumes that students with disabilities will be held to the same state standards as students without disabilities. It expects that special education and related services will be closely aligned with the general curriculum and that students with disabilities will master that curriculum and graduate with their peers without disabilities.

After years of minimal improvement in students' reading ability, the country took a new look at reading. Reid Lyon led research efforts at the National Institutes of Health that identified phonological awareness as a necessary component of beginning reading (Lyon & Chabra, 1996). Oral language has long been recognized as a necessary precursor to the development of written language (reference). Throughout the country, public school systems are assessing young children's phonological awareness skills and providing phonological awareness development and remediation activities.

With intensive backgrounds in phonology and language, speech-language pathologists can be vital participants in the academic achievement of children in public education. Speech-language pathologists' skills in language and knowledge of its influence on curriculum and instruction can be useful in curriculum design and development, especially in the area of English/language arts. Speech-language pathologists' knowledge of phonetics, phonology, and language enables them to work cooperatively with pre-kindergarten and primary teachers as they help young children to develop phonological awareness skills. The future appears to be one of opportunity for public school speech-language pathologists. Yet, if speech-language pathologists are not prepared to participate, will the future be one in which reading specialists and teachers assume part of the role of school speech-language pathologists?

The nation's intense focus on student achievement may cause parents to question the value of removing their children from the regular education classroom for services. Such removal will reduce the child's opportunity to master the material in the core academic areas. The majority of speech-language services are provided in a pull-out model (78%), whereas only a small portion of these services use the classroom-based model (13%) or collaborative consultation model (5%) (American Speech-Language-Hearing Association, 1996). This approach may no longer be sufficient to meet students' needs. The future is more positive for clinicians who work collaboratively with general and special education teachers, integrating speech-language services with the classroom communication demands. Students will progress more rapidly and speech-language pathologists will find themselves valued for the expertise they lend to public education. Blosser and Kratcoski (1997) remind speech-language pathologists that although they have the expertise for identifying the language strengths and needs, there are multiple providers, activities and contexts in which communication can be developed. Their PAC (provider, activity, and contexts) model can be a tool for speech-language pathologists to use to more effectively meet their clients needs. By identifying those persons (providers) with whom the child interacts (i.e., teachers, aides, parents) and the activities (classroom presentation, conversation at home), and contexts (classroom, church/synagogue) speech-language pathologists can identify the vast number of opportunities available for facilitating effective communication skills. The PAC model continues with identifying barriers to effective use of other providers and vehicles for resolving those barriers. By utilizing this model, speech-language pathologists will be better equipped to meet students' needs in school as demanded for reducing the time out of the classroom increases.

Accountability

The educational reform movement also includes high expectations for accountability. Parents, employers, taxpayers, and politicians demand that schools demonstrate improvement in students' academic performance.

The IDEA Amendments of 1997 also raised expectations for accountability in special education and related services. Parents are to be informed of their child's progress on the same schedule as parents of students without disabilities. Further, aggregate student performance is to be reported to the public. Educators are expected to provide data to demonstrate student achievement. This recent emphasis on reporting results is likely to become a fixture in public education.

Do speech-language pathologists have the data necessary to prove the difference their services make with young children? Efforts by Swigert, Gallagher and others (Gallagher, Swigert, & Baum, 1998) have enabled ASHA to gather outcomes data. Although this data collection began in health care, the issues are equally relevant in educational settings (see also Chapter 2). Public school speech-language pathologists must participate in the development of a treatment outcomes database. Through their involvement, speech-language pathologists can anticipate answering questions such as the following in the coming years:

- If young children with language impairments receive speech-language pathology services, will they learn how to read faster or better?
- What will the effect of services be on academic achievement?
- What will be the effect of speech-language pathology services on special education eligibility?
- What will be the effect of speech-language pathology services on social interactions and self-esteem?
- What part of speech-language pathology services can be effectively provided by others, for example by kindergarten teachers or teachers of students with learning disabilities?
- How much intervention is necessary to ameliorate a communication impairment in a kindergarten child?

Reliance on instinct, clinical intuition, and triennial assessments is not sufficient for documentation of students' progress. Public school speech-language pathologists must integrate data collection into their daily routine. Without such data, speech-language pathologists cannot demonstrate their influence on children's achievement, and their influence in the future will be diminished. Armed with data, speech-language pathologists' future is more positive because they can convince fellow educators and policy makers that speech-language pathologists are vital members of the public education team.

School Safety

School safety issues have transformed the nation's schools. School resource officers and security measures (such as cameras and search dogs) are now commonplace in suburban and urban schools, as well as rural schools. Strict codes of conduct are used to maintain discipline. What is the role of speech-language pathologists with respect to school safety? One essential feature of violence prevention is effective communication. Students with semantic-pragmatic deficits generally have difficulty communicating effectively with peers, recognizing differences in communication patterns, expressing themselves clearly, and recognizing and repairing communication breakdowns. In addition to working with students with communication impairments, speech-language pathologists who are skilled in working with adolescents can be valuable team members in schools that use conflict mediation. Conflict mediation is a valuable technique that enables school officials to teach students methods of resolving conflict without resorting to violence (Institute for Conflict Analysis and Resolution, 1997). These methods rely on effective listening and understanding skills as well as effective expression. Improving students' communication skills can help maintain school safety and a more positive school climate. What can we predict of the future? Increased focus on violence prevention is a certainty. Whether speech-language pathologists will lend their expertise is up to them.

CULTURAL-LINGUISTIC DIVERSITY

The United States is becoming increasingly heterogeneous. Cultural and linguistic minorities currently represent one-fourth of the U.S. population. By 2050, Native Americans, Asians, African Americans, and Hispanics will account for approximately half of the U.S. population. Nearly 1 in 10 people currently residing in the United States was born somewhere else, and many of these persons speak a language other than English as their native language. The concentration of minority enrollments in public schools is greatest in the nation's largest urban school systems (Power-deFur, 1995a; Goldberg, 1997a).

Given the high academic standards in English in our nation's public schools, students from culturally-linguistically diverse backgrounds may have difficulty with the language demands of academic instruction. In general, academic achievement and high school completion rates are lower, and dropout rates and incarceration rates are higher for culturally-linguistically different groups than for the general population. What can we predict about the future academic performance of culturally-linguistically diverse students? Internal scans inform us that speech-language pathologists are currently not completely competent to treat individuals from racial and ethnic minority groups (Uffen, 1998). What are the consequences of not becoming more competent?

Educators and clinicians from the majority culture generally work with culturally-linguistically different students. Although many clinicians from the majority culture exhibit cultural competency, there is a tremendous lack of sufficient culturally-linguistically diverse professionals in the field. Expanding our own cultural competency and promoting the entrance of students from culturally-linguistically diverse populations into the speech-language pathology profession can positively influence the future. Without such efforts, there will likely be continued disparity in the academic performance of the majority population and culturally-linguistically diverse populations.

The increasing cultural-linguistic diversity of the U.S. population leads to further predictions. The English language is one of four languages that are the official or preferred language in all but 70 of the world's 200–plus nations (the others are Arabic, French, and Spanish). English seems destined to dominate the world as more people study English as a second language than any other tongue. However, nonnative English speakers outnumber native speakers by four to one (Jennings, 1998). This phenomenon will result in a future in which the English language evolves with new vocabulary that is based on the native languages of the nonnative English speakers. These changes will be in addition to those changes in the language due to advances in science and technology and societal changes. As language experts, speech-language pathologists can anticipate these changes, stay abreast of the dynamic nature of the language, and integrate new vocabulary and language usages into their work.

SUPPLY AND DEMAND OF SPEECH-LANGUAGE PATHOLOGISTS

External scans suggest that the number of speech-language pathology positions in public education and health care will continue to expand into the next century due to the aging population, the improved lifesaving techniques for newborns, and the anticipated growth in the public school population. Internal scans inform us that we can anticipate retirement of many speech-language pathologists (Power-deFur, 1996). The result may be a demand for speech-language pathologists that exceeds supply.

Given the significant changes in health care reimbursement in the late 20th century (Davolt, 1998; Spracher, 1998), the near future provides an opportunity for schools to hire speech-language pathologists who are moving out of health care settings. Public schools throughout the country will continue to seek speech-language pathologists with master's degrees and ASHA certification. Clinicians who are bilingual, computer savvy, and experienced in working with clients with dysphagia, or experienced in working with clients needing assistive technology will be the most sought after professionals.

Internal and external scans also suggest increased demand for speech-language pathology support personnel (Kimbarow, 1997). Whether they use support personnel to assist with clerical duties or clinical duties, speech-language pathologists will need to learn delegation and supervisory skills. Clinicians must be able to delineate between the tasks that require the skills of a qualified speech-language pathologist and those that require trained support personnel. The future will also bring opportunities for training support personnel. Speech-language pathologists must be involved in all aspects of the growth of support personnel—including the delegation of duties, training, and supervision. In this future scenario, it is better that speech-language pathologists retain their involvement than walk away from it and let other professionals step in to these roles.

TECHNOLOGY AND THE INFORMATION AGE

The information explosion is stunning in its impact. In highly technical jobs, as much as half of the knowledge base becomes obsolete in three to five years. There is more information in one edition of the Sunday *New York Times* than individuals encountered in an entire lifetime in the 1700s (Power-deFur, 1995a). The body of knowledge will have doubled four times between 1988 and 2000 (Cetron, 1990). Graduates in the year 2000 will have been exposed that year to more information than their grandparents were in a lifetime (Cetron, 1988).

How can clinicians possibly be able to handle all the information bombarding them? Improved personal information management skills will be necessary. Because we cannot retain all the new information, we must know how to access the necessary information and know when to refer to a specialist. Technology has brought this expansion of information and provides tools for managing the information. Consider that all the technology we work with today represents 1% of the technology that will be available in the year 2050 (Power-deFur, 1995a). With middle school and even elementary school students developing Web pages and using databases, what will be the role of the school speech-language pathologist without information technology skills?

External scans inform us that there will be fewer jobs requiring manual labor and more jobs relying on sophisticated management of information and data. As speech-language pathologists prepare students for the workforce of tomorrow, they must remain abreast of the language and communication demands of that future workforce.

The expansion of electronic communication will likely influence the art of communication. Telephone conversations and conference calls are not the same as dialogues in person. Electronic communication is not the same as oral communication. Yet, consumer demand for speed and instant gratification continues to expand, increasing our use of technology for communication. Could the art of face-to-face communication become lost in the computer age? Some have noted "a disturbing trend in human communication, namely, the demise of decency" (Werven, 1996). Has this trend been influenced by electronic communication methods? How will it change in the future? Moreover, what, if any, is the role of the speech-language pathologist? As communication professionals, speech-language pathologists should observe and evaluate the changing nature of human communication to determine trends. With such study, speech-language pathologists can influence the changes as necessary.

TECHNOLOGY, SPEECH-LANGUAGE CASELOADS, AND SERVICE DELIVERY

Public school speech-language pathology caseloads have changed a great deal over the last half-century. We have moved from speech teachers to "full-service" communication specialists. Caseloads have become more diverse as speech-language pathologists have begun serving students with neurological impairments, students with dysphagia, and students requiring augmentative communication. It is not hard to predict that there will be additional changes in the future. What will be the nature of the changes in caseloads? How will technology play a role?

Scientists will discover the genetic link to many human behaviors and traits as they map the human genome (Power-deFur, 1995a). Recently, researchers have uncovered evidence for a genetic link to stuttering (Vairi, 1998). Further links between communication disorders and genetics are anticipated. Will genetic engineering replace speech-language pathologists in the future? Not likely. Nevertheless, the future will require speech-language pathologists to have knowledge of the relationship between genetics and communication disorders and tailor the intervention appropriately.

It was no so long ago that the concept of telemedicine challenged our sense of ethics. How could a professional ethically provide services to a client without being in the same location? Advances in technology now enable health care professionals to provide services to sites that are so remote or so poorly accessible that specialists cannot be on site (Goldberg, 1997b). Will the technology supporting telemedicine have an impact on public education? Most assuredly. Higher education has been using this technology to provide coursework via distance for decades. Many public schools have used such distance education to provide advanced classes to students in remote locations. Can speech-language pathologists apply this technology to assessment and intervention with students possessing communication impairments? In fact, there are numerous possibilities for harnessing new technologies to benefit these students.

Interactive multimedia is fast becoming a valuable tool of education. In 1988, Cetron predicted that by the year 2000 "computer-aided learning programs . . . will begin to replace some kinds of textbooks as well" (Cetron, 1990). However, researchers have found that the realism of high-tech simulations does not necessarily or consistently translate into learning that is more effective and better retained. Consider speech-language pathologists' past experience with drill work and clinicians' frustration with the inability of students to "generalize" newly acquired skills to other settings. Could the use of technology for instruction also be prone to the same problem? Clinicians should not revisit past mistakes by overrelying on computer technology for communication intervention. It is important for speech-language pathologists to harness this emerging trend and apply it in such a way that it enables students to learn new skills and readily apply them in functional ways.

Technology has enabled persons to receive cochlear implants at younger and younger ages. Increasingly, parents are expecting public schools to provide services to children with a cochlear implants—services that emphasize auditory training, oral language, and speech production. More students with cochlear implants will be in our public schools in the future. A change in deaf education programs can be predicted. Speech-language pathologists, deaf educators, and audiologists will need to be prepared to meet the auditory training and oral communication needs of these children.

Advances in medical procedures and technology will allow more children to survive prematurity, traumatic brain injury, and other life-threatening events. These children have a right to a public education and will challenge school districts, educators, and therapists. Students who are medically fragile will have a host of medical needs to be attended to in schools. Speech-language pathologists can anticipate working with students with dysphagia and those who need ventilators and other medical equipment. To work with such children, speech-language pathologists must remain up-to-date in their knowledge, skills, and abilities, for the benefit of the students, to abide by the ASHA Code of Ethics and to reduce potential liability to the school district (Power-deFur, in press).

The anticipated increase in the number of medically fragile students in public schools may also increase the demands for assistive technology. IDEA 97 directs Individualized Education Program (IEP) teams to consider assistive technology needs for all children who are eligible for special education and related services. Speech-language pathologists with skills in assistive technology, especially augmentative and alternative communication (AAC) devices, will be in high demand. Not only will speech-language pathologists need to be sophisticated in electronic and computer gadgetry, they also will need expertise in addressing the effect of augmentative communication on language and literacy. How is social interaction that is based on electronic communication, either by an AAC device or e-mail, different from social interaction that is based on oral communication? Does reliance on electronic modes of communication affect literacy skills? Can children communicating electronically develop the phonological awareness skills that are necessary precursors to learning to read? These questions require the attention of researchers and clinicians.

THIRD-PARTY REIMBURSEMENT AND PUBLIC SCHOOLS

The public attitude toward taxes and the role of government has resulted in tax reforms throughout the country. One of the byproducts is the increased scrutiny of public dollars funding education. Policymakers at local, state, and national levels frequently criticize the high cost of special education. Despite the mandate to provide special education and related services, it will be necessary to seek additional sources of funding (Jones & Power-deFur, 1997).

IDEA permits school systems to access both public and private insurance to pay for services. Because speech-language pathology is a discipline that straddles education and health care, speech-language services provided in schools can be billed to third-party payers. Since the late 1980s, Medicaid funding has been accessed to support services offered in schools for students eligible for both special education and Medicaid. Medicaid paperwork requirements are viewed as onerous, especially when added to IDEA documentation requirements. In states that employ speech-language pathologists who do not meet the highest qualifications (master's degree in speech-language pathology and ASHA certification), there will be clinicians who Medicaid will not recognized as a qualified provider. Further, there are no restrictions on the use of Medicaid funds, so dollars generated by speech-language pathologists providing speech therapy to students eligible for Medicaid can be used elsewhere in the school district. The incentive for school districts to use Medicaid funding is great.

The future will see increased efforts by school districts to pursue Medicaid and private insurance to offset some of the public dollars supporting special education. To have an influence, public school speech-language pathologists will need to develop the knowledge and skills in third-party reimbursement previously limited to their colleagues in health care settings.

POSITIONING FOR THE FUTURE

The future of public school speech-language pathology will certainly bring change. It is human nature to resist change. Change naturally raises three areas of concern: Who will create the change? What is the nature of the change? How will the change occur? The changes that are most resisted are those that are imposed on people. Speech-language pathologists can choose whether to be involved in the future changes and influence the effect of the changes on their profession and their consumers. In this way, speech-lnaguage pathologists will have a small ownership in the change itself. Consider the following suggestions for being prepared for the future:

- Broaden your knowledge of education standards and curriculum, especially oral language.
- Learn more about the beginning reading process and the relationship between reading and oral language.
- Participate in the development of academic standards and curriculum at the school, district, state, or national level.
- Partner with parents, reading teachers, special education teachers, regular education teachers, vocational education teachers, principals, school safety specialists, school nurses, occupational therapists, physical therapists, and support personnel to meet the communication needs of students.
- View cross-disciplinary service delivery as an opportunity to demonstrate your value to other professionals.
- Update your knowledge on dysphagia.
- Remain current in technology, especially information management and augmentative communication.
- Maintain an in-depth understanding of the science underlying professional practices so that you are viewed by your education colleagues as a coprofessional, not a technician.
- Develop a greater understanding of the heterogeneous nature of American cultures. Develop skills in working with multicultural populations.
- Master a language other than English.
- Monitor your own performance.
- Gather data on your students' performance and the results of your interventions.
- Use national outcomes data to demonstrate the need for and to project the length of services.
- Stay abreast of the communication demands of the workforce.
- Pursue opportunities for leadership in administrative positions and policy-making positions.
- Stay current in your knowledge of language as it evolves.
- Choose to become involved in the future. Observe trends. Anticipate results. Stay involved and active. Let the future become yours to influence, rather than influencing you.

REFERENCES

American Speech-Language-Hearing Association. (1996). *Survey of speech-language pathology services in school-based settings*. Rockville, MD: Author.

Blosser, J.L., & Kratcoski, A. (1997). PACS: A framework for determining appropriate service delivery options. *Language, Speech, and Hearing Services in Schools, 28*, 99–107.

Cetron, M.J. (1990). Class of 2000. In E. Cornish (Ed), *The 1990s and Beyond* (pp. 41–47). Bethesda, MD: World Future Society.

Davolt, S. (1998, December 22). Providers adapt to new Medicare payment plan. *ASHA Leader, 3*, 24, 1, 4.

Elam, S.M., Rose, L.C., & Gallup, A.M. (1994, September). The 26th annual Phi Delta Kappa/Gallup Poll of the public's attitudes toward the public schools. *Phi Delta Kappan,* 41–56.

Gallagher, T.M., Swigert, N.B., & Baum, H.M. (1998). Collecting outcomes data in schools: Needs and challenges. *Language, Speech, and Hearing Services in Schools, 29*, 250–256.

Gelatt, J. (1994). *Managerial planning and competitive strategies*. College Park, MD: University of Maryland, University College.

Goldberg, B., (1997a). Tailoring to fit: Altering our approach to multicultural populations. *Asha, 39*,(2), 22–28.

Goldberg, B. (1997b). Linking up with telehealth. *Asha, 39*,(3), 26–31.

Herer, G. (1989). *Major trends affecting the future of communication disorders: A report of the ASHA Executive Board colloquia on the future*. Rockville, MD: American Speech-Language-Hearing Association.

Institute for Conflict Analysis and Resolution. (1997). *Understanding intergroup conflict in schools*. Fairfax, VA: George Mason University.

Jennings, L. (1998). Futurespeak. *Asha, 40*,(1), 8.

Jones, L., & Power-deFur. (1997). Financing inclusive education programs. In L. Power-deFur & F. Orelove (Eds.). *Inclusive education: Practical implementation of the least restrictive environment* (pp. 63–73). Gaithersburg, MD: Aspen Publishers, Inc.

Kimbarow, M. (1997). Ahead of the curve: Improving service with speech-language pathology assistants. *Asha, 39*,(3), 41–44.

Lyon, G.R., & Chabra, V. (1996). The current state of science and the future of specific reading disability. *Mental Retardation and Developmental Disabilities Research Reviews, 2,* 2–9.

McLaughlin, M.J., Nolet, V., Rhim, L.M., & Henderson, K. (1999, January/February). Integrating standards: Including all students. *Teaching Exceptional Children*, 60–64.

Montgomery, J.K., & Herer, G. (1994). Future watch: Our schools in the 21st century. *Language, Speech and Hearing Services in Schools, 25*, 130–135.

Power-deFur, L. (In press). Serving students with dysphagia in the schools. *Language, Speech, and Hearing Services in Schools*.

Power-deFur, L. (1995a). Thinking about your future. Paper presented at the Annual Convention of the American Speech-Language-Hearing Association, Orlando, FL.

Power-deFur, L. (1996). Membership–The baby boomers grow up and other challenges. Paper presented at the meeting of ASHA Legislative Council, Seattle, WA.

Spracher, M. (1998, December 22). As $1,500 cap arrives, need for advocacy grows. *ASHA Leader, 3*, 24, 1.

Uffen, E. (1998). Where the jobs are: Keeping an eye on the future. *Asha, 40*, 25–28.

Vairi, E. (1998). Is the basis of stuttering genetic? *Asha, 40*, 29–32.

Werven, G. (1996). (Un)civilized speech: Should ASHA care? *Asha, 38*, 5.

World Future Society. (1993). *The art of forecasting*. Bethesda, MD: Author.

SUGGESTED READINGS

American Speech-Language-Hearing Association. (1994). *Trends and issues in school reform and their effects on speech-language pathologists, audiologists, and students with communication disorders. A technical report prepared by the Ad Hoc Committee on Changes in Education Policies and Practices*. Rockville, MD: Author.

Geffner, D. (1997). Growing the field. Who will teach future generations? *Asha, 39*, 3, 37–42.

Goldberg, B. (1996). Imagining tomorrow: What's ahead for our professions. *Asha, 38*,(3), 22–28.

Power-deFur, L. (1995b). *The workforce of the 21st century: ASHA future watch. A report of the Long Range Strategic Planning Board*. Rockville, MD: American Speech-Language-Hearing Association.

Tsantis, L., & Keefe, D. (1996). Reinventing education. *Asha, 38*, 4, 38–42.

Index

A

B

E

H

I

L

M

Q

R

S

T

U

V

W